APPROXIMATE EQUIVALENTS FOR METRIC, APOTHECARY, AND HOUSEHOLD WEIGHTS AND VOLUMES

Approximate Equivalents for Weight

Metric	Apothecary
1 kg (1000 g)	2.2 lb
1 g (1000 mg)	15 gr
60 mg	1 gr

Approximate Equivalents for Volume

Metric	Apothecary	Household
4000 mL	1 gal (4 qt)	
1 L (1000 mL)	1 qt (2 pt)	
500 mL	1 pt (16 fl oz)	
240 mL	8 oz	1 cup
30 mL	1 oz (8 dr)	2 tbsp
15 mL	½ oz (4 dr)	1 tbsp (3 tsp)
5 mL	1 dr (60 M)	1 tsp (60 gtt)
1 mL	15 M	15 gtt
	1 M	1 gtt

CELSIUS AND FAHRENHEIT TEMPERATURE EQUIVALENTS

** Conversion Chart **		
Celsius	to	Fahrenheit
35.0		95.0
35.5		95.9
36.0		96.8
36.5		97.7
37.0		98.6
37.5		99.5
38.0		100.4
38.5		101.3
39.0		102.2
39.5		103.1
40.0		104.0
40.5		104.9
41.0		105.8
41.5		106.7
42.0		107.6

To convert from Fahrenheit to Celsius:
$$°C = (°F - 32) \div 1.8$$

To convert from Celsius to Fahrenheit:
$$°F = °C \times 1.8 + 32$$

$°C$ = temperature in degrees Celsius
$°F$ = temperature in degrees Fahrenheit

Clinical Calculations
Made Easy

FOURTH EDITION

Clinical Calculations Made Easy

Solving Problems Using Dimensional Analysis

Gloria P. Craig, RN, MSN, EdD
Associate Professor
South Dakota State University
College of Nursing
Brookings, South Dakota

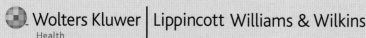 Wolters Kluwer | Lippincott Williams & Wilkins
Health
Philadelphia • Baltimore • New York • London
Buenos Aires • Hong Kong • Sydney • Tokyo

Acquisitions Editor: Hillarie Surrena
Managing Editor: Helen Kogut
Editorial Assistant: Elizabeth Harris
Senior Production Editor: Mary Kinsella
Director of Nursing Production: Helen Ewan
Senior Managing Editor / Production: Erika Kors
Design Coordinator: Holly Reid McLaughlin
Interior Design: Lisa Delgado
Cover Design: Bess Kiethas
Art Director, Illustration: Brett MacNaughton
Manufacturing Coordinator: Karin Duffield
Indexer: Angie Allen
Compositor: Circle Graphics

Fourth Edition

9 8 7 6 5 4 3 2 1

Printed in China

Library of Congress Cataloging-in-Publication Data

Craig, Gloria P., 1949-
  Clinical calculations made easy : solving problems using dimensional analysis / Gloria P. Craig. — 4th ed.
       p. ; cm.
  Includes bibliographical references and index.
  ISBN 978-0-7817-6385-1 (alk. paper)
  1. Pharmaceutical arithmetic. 2. Dimensional analysis. 3. Nursing—Mathematics. I. Title.
  [DNLM: 1. Pharmaceutical Preparations—administration & dosage. 2. Mathematics. 3. Nurses' Instruction. 4. Problem Solving.
5. Problems and Exercises.   QV 748 C886ca 2009]
  RS57.C73 2009
  615'.14—dc22

                                                                        2007042536

Care has been taken to confirm the accuracy of the information presented and to describe generally accepted practices. However, the authors, editors, and publisher are not responsible for errors or omissions or for any consequences from application of the information in this book and make no warranty, expressed or implied, with respect to the currency, completeness, or accuracy of the contents of the publication. Application of this information in a particular situation remains the professional responsibility of the practitioner; the clinical treatments described and recommended may not be considered absolute and universal recommendations.

The authors, editors, and publisher have exerted every effort to ensure that drug selection and dosage set forth in this text are in accordance with the current recommendations and practice at the time of publication. However, in view of ongoing research, changes in government regulations, and the constant flow of information relating to drug therapy and drug reactions, the reader is urged to check the package insert for each drug for any change in indications and dosage and for added warnings and precautions. This is particularly important when the recommended agent is a new or infrequently employed drug.

Some drugs and medical devices presented in this publication have Food and Drug Administration (FDA) clearance for limited use in restricted research settings. It is the responsibility of the health care provider to ascertain the FDA status of each drug or device planned for use in his or her clinical practice.

Reviewers

Teresa Aprigliano, EdD, RN
Associate Professor, Director
Molloy College
Rockville Centre, New York

Patricia Ann Dudley, MSN, RN, CRNP
Nursing Faculty
University of Alabama at Birmingham
Birmingham, Alabama

Sharon Koval Falkenstern, PhD, CRNP, PNP-C
Instructor, Family Nurse Practitioner Program Coordinator
Pennsylvania State University
University Park, Pennsylvania

Barbara J. Hoerst, PhD, RN
Assistant Professor
La Salle University
Philadelphia, Pennsylvania

Cathy Malone, MSN, BSN, RN
Assistant Professor
University of North Alabama
Florence, Alabama

Anna Sanford, MSN, APRN, BC
Associate Professor
Northern Michigan University
Marquette, Michigan

Cynthia L. Terry, MSN, RN, CCRN
Professor
Lehigh Carbon Community College
Schnecksville, Pennsylvania

Ina E. Warboys, MS, RN
Clinical Assistant Professor
University of Alabama in Huntsville
Huntsville, Alabama

Loretta L. White, DNS, RN
Assistant Professor
Indiana State University
Terre Haute, Indiana

Rosemary Wittstadt, EdD, RN
Adjunct Professor
Howard Community College
Columbia, Maryland

Many people experience stumbling blocks calculating math problems because of a lack of mathematical ability or associated "math anxiety." Even people with strong math skills often set up medication problems incorrectly, putting the patient at an increased risk for incorrect dosages and the ensuing consequences. However, dosage calculation need not be difficult if you use a problem-solving method that is easy to understand and to implement.

As a student, I experienced anxiety related to poor mathematical abilities and consequently had difficulty with medication calculations. However, a friend introduced me to a problem-solving method that was easy to visualize. By using this method, I was able to easily understand medication problems and thereby avoid the stumbling blocks that I had experienced with other methods of dosage calculations. Later, as a practicing nurse and nursing instructor, I realized that many of my colleagues and students shared my experience with "math anxiety," so I began sharing this problem-solving method with them.

During my baccalaureate nursing education, this problem-solving method became my teaching plan. During my master's education, it became my research. During my doctoral education, it became my dissertation. Now, I would like to share this method with anyone who ever believed that they were mathematically "challenged" or trembled at the thought of solving a medication problem.

The method, called dimensional analysis (also known as factor-label method or conversion-factor method), is a systematic, straightforward approach to setting up and solving problems that require conversions. It is a way of thinking about problems that can be used when two quantities are directly proportional to each other, but one needs to be converted using a conversion factor in order for the problem to be solved.

Dimensional Analysis as a Teaching Tool

Dimensional analysis empowers the learner to solve a variety of medication problems using just one problem-solving method. Research has shown that students experience less frustration and create fewer *medication errors* if one problem-solving method is used to solve *all* medication problems. As a method of reducing errors and improving calculation *abilities,* dimensional analysis has many possibilities. Whether it is used in practice or education, it is a strong approach when the goals are improving medication dosage-calculation skills, reducing medication errors, and improving patient safety. Ultimately, this improved methodology has the potential to reduce the medication errors that occur within the discipline of nursing.

Dimensional analysis helps the learner see and understand the significance of the whole process, since it focuses on how to learn, rather than what to learn. It provides a framework for understanding the principles of the problem-solving method and supports the critical thinking process. It helps the learner to organize and evaluate data, and to avoid errors in setting up problems. Dimensional analysis thus supports the conceptual mastery and higher-level thinking skills that have become the core of curricula at all levels of nursing education.

Organization of the Text

This text uses the simple-to-complex approach in teaching students clinical calculations and is, therefore, divided into four sections.

Section 1: Clinical Calculations

Chapter 1 provides an arithmetic pretest to help gauge the amount of time a student will need to spend reviewing the basic arithmetic skills presented in this chapter.

Chapter 2 reviews systems of measurement, common equivalents, calculating patient intake and output, and converting standard time and military time.

Chapter 3 introduces the student to dimensional analysis and uses common equivalents to help the student practice problem solving with this new method.

Chapter 4 builds on the previous chapter by introducing one-factor conversions.

Chapter 5 continues the growth process by presenting two-factor conversions.

Chapter 6 completes the student's understanding of clinical calculations by introducing three-factor conversions.

Section 2: Practice Problems

Section 2 allows the student the opportunity to refine the skills presented in section 1 by providing additional one-, two-, and three-factor practice problems followed by comprehensive questions to ensure accurate understanding of clinical calculations.

Section 3: Case Studies

Section 3 helps the student relate dosage calculations to real clinical situations. Thirty-five case studies that are related to different fields of nursing are included in this section.

Section 4: Comprehensive Post-Test

Section 4 contains a post-test of 20 questions allowing the instructor to assess the student's mastery of solving clinical calculations using dimensional analysis. The answers to these questions as well as additional post-tests are available to instructors on thePoint.

Special Features

Each chapter in *Section 1* contains *numerous* **Examples** with detailed explanations. **Thinking It Through** provides additional explanations to help students more fully understand complex topics. *In-chapter* **Exercises** occur after the presentation and explanation of each new concept, providing an opportunity for the student to gain ability and confidence in the material before proceeding to the next concept. Additional **Practice Problems** are provided at the end of the chapter so that students can practice the skills and assess areas where more review may be necessary. An **Answer Key** for all Exercises and Practice Problems is also located at the end of each chapter. Additionally, a **Post-Test,** designed so that students can tear it out of the book and hand it in to their instructor, appears at the end of each chapter. The answers for all Post-Tests are also available to instructors on thePoint.

In addition:

- **Actual drug labels** are liberally used throughout the text to provide the student with clinically realistic examples.

- A special feature, **Preventing Medication Errors,** helps identify key concepts necessary for avoiding clinical calculation errors.

- A special icon identifying **pediatric medication problems** allows students and teachers to quickly find all pediatric problems in the text.

New to This Edition

The fourth edition provides many more opportunities for students to practice their skills. **More problems** have been added throughout the text and all problems have been updated to follow **guidelines from the Institute for Safe Medication Practices. Calculation of intake and output** and converting **standard time and military time** are included to aid students in learning accurate medical recording. **Ten new case studies** *including pediatric problems* have also been added as well as a **new Comprehensive Post-Test.**

Resources on thePoint

thePoint (http://thepoint.lww.com), a trademark of Wolters Kluwer Health, is a web-based course and content management system providing every resource that instructors and students need in one easy-to-use site. Advanced technology and superior content combine at thePoint to allow instructors to design and deliver on-line and off-line courses, maintain grades and class rosters, and communicate with students.

Instructors will also find

- Answer keys for all Post-Tests
- Instructor's Manual
- PowerPoint presentations

Students can visit thePoint to access supplemental multimedia resources to enhance their learning experience, download content, upload assignments, and join an on-line study group.

Also available to students are

- Additional practice problems
- Additional post-tests

By using this text and all of its resources, it is my hope that this fourth edition will help students find that clinical calculation can indeed be made easy using dimensional analysis.

Gloria P. Craig

Acknowledgments

There are many people who have assisted me with my professional growth and development, including:

Pauline Callahan, who believed that I would be a great nurse and nursing instructor when I could not believe in myself.

Jackie Kehm, who introduced me to dimensional analysis and helped me pass the medication module that I was sure would be my stumbling block.

Dr. Sandra L. Sellers, for her expertise and guidance throughout the process of writing my thesis and dissertation and her encouragement to write a textbook.

Margaret Cooper, for her friendship and editing support throughout the writing of this textbook.

My students, colleagues, and reviewers, for helping me develop my abilities to explain and teach the problem-solving method of dimensional analysis.

The numerous pharmaceutical companies listed throughout this book that supplied medication labels and gave permission for the labels to be included in this textbook.

The faculty at South Dakota State University, College of Nursing, for allowing dimensional analysis to be integrated into the curriculum as the problem-solving method for medication calculation.

The Lippincott editorial and production teams, for all of their hard work: **Hillarie Surrena,** Senior Acquisitions Editor; **Helen Kogut,** Managing Editor; **Mary Kinsella,** Senior Production Editor; and **Holly Reid McLaughlin,** Design Coordinator.

To these people and many more, I would like to express my sincere appreciation for their mentoring, guidance, support, and encouragement that have helped to turn a dream into a reality.

This fourth edition of my text is dedicated to my children, **Lori (and her husband, Michael) and Randy (and his wife Samantha),** and to my granddaughters, **Zoë, Ava, and Lily.**

Contents

Chapter 1 Pre-Test: Arithmetic Review

Name _____   **Date** _____

Converting Between Arabic Numbers and Roman Numerals

1. 7   = _____

2. XI   = _____

3. 17   = _____

4. XVI = _____

Multiplying and Dividing Fractions

5. $\dfrac{2}{8} \times \dfrac{2}{2} =$

6. $\dfrac{2}{5} \div \dfrac{1}{10} =$

7. $\dfrac{2}{6} \times \dfrac{1}{2} =$

8. $\dfrac{1}{3} \div \dfrac{3}{9} =$

9. $\dfrac{3}{4} \times \dfrac{2}{3} =$

10. $\dfrac{2}{4} \div \dfrac{1}{2} =$

Converting Fractions to Decimals

11. $\dfrac{4}{8} =$

12. $\dfrac{2}{6} =$

13. $\dfrac{5}{9} =$

14. $\dfrac{1}{4} =$

Multiplying and Dividing Decimals

15. $2.75 \times 1.25 =$

16. $0.25 \div 0.4 =$

17. $4.50 \times 0.75 =$

18. $10.50 \div 4.5 =$

19. $1.2 \times 2 =$

20. $1.5 \div 0.75 =$

CHAPTER 1

Arithmetic Review

Objectives

After completing this chapter, you will successfully be able to:

1. **Express Arabic numbers as Roman numerals.**
2. **Express Roman numerals as Arabic numbers.**
3. **Identify the numerator and denominator in a fraction.**
4. **Multiply and divide fractions.**
5. **Multiply and divide decimals.**
6. **Convert fractions to decimals.**

Outline

Every nurse must know and practice the six rights of medication administration including the

1. Right drug
2. Right dose
3. Right route
4. Right time
5. Right patient
6. Right documentation

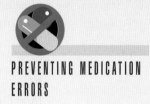

PREVENTING MEDICATION ERRORS

Although the right drug, route, time, patient, and documentation may be readily identified, the right dose requires **arithmetic skills** that may be difficult for you. This chapter reviews the basic arithmetic skills (multiplication and division) **necessary for calculating** medication dosage problems using the problem-solving method of dimensional analysis. Calculating the **right dose** of medication to be administered to a patient is one of the first steps toward preventing **medication errors.**

■ ARABIC NUMBERS AND ROMAN NUMERALS

Most medication dosages are ordered by the physician or the nurse practitioner in the metric and household systems for weights and measures using the Arabic number system with symbols called **digits** (ie, 1, 2, 3, 4, 5). Occasionally, orders are received in the apothecaries' system of weights and measures using the Roman numeral system with numbers represented by **symbols** (ie, I, V, X). The Roman numeral system uses seven basic symbols, and various combinations of these symbols represent all numbers in the Arabic number system.

Table 1.1 includes the seven basic Roman numerals and the corresponding Arabic numbers.

The combination of Roman numeral symbols is based on three specific principles:

1. Symbols are used to construct a number, but no symbol may be used more than three times. The exception is the symbol for five (V), which is used only once because there is a symbol for 10 (X) and a combination of symbols for 15 (XV).

EXAMPLE 1.1

III = (1 + 1 + 1) = 3
XXX = (10 + 10 + 10) = 30

2. When symbols of lesser value follow symbols of greater value, they are *added* to construct a number.

EXAMPLE 1.2

VIII = (5 + 3) = 8
XVII = (10 + 5 + 1 + 1) = 17

3. When symbols of greater value follow symbols of lesser value, those of lesser value are *subtracted* from those of higher value to construct a number.

EXAMPLE 1.3

IV = (5 - 1) = 4
IX = (10 - 1) = 9

■ TABLE 1.1	Seven Basic Roman Numerals
ROMAN NUMERALS	**ARABIC NUMBERS**
I	1
V	5
X	10
L	50
C	100
D	500
M	1000

Exercise 1.1	**Arabic Numbers and Roman Numerals**
	(See page 23 for answers)

Express the following Arabic numbers as Roman numerals.

1. 1 = _____

2. 2 = _____

3. 3 = _____

4. 4 = _____

5. 5 = _____

6. 6 = _____

7. 7 = _____

8. 8 = _____

9. 9 = _____

10. 10 = _____

11. 11 = _____

12. 12 = _____

13. 13 = _____

14. 14 = _____

15. 15 = _____

16. 16 = _____

17. 17 = _____

18. 18 = _____

19. 19 = _____

20. 20 = _____

Although medication orders rarely involve Roman numerals higher than 20, for additional practice, express the following Arabic numbers as Roman numerals.

21. 43 = _____

22. 24 = _____

23. 55 = _____

24. 32 = _____

25. 102 = _____

26. 150 = _____

(Exercise continues on page 8)

27. 75 = _____

28. 92 = _____

29. 64 = _____

30. 69 = _____

Express the following Roman numerals as Arabic numbers.

31. II   = _____

32. IV   = _____

33. VI   = _____

34. X   = _____

35. VIII = _____

36. XIX = _____

37. XX   = _____

38. XVIII = _____

39. I   = _____

40. XV   = _____

41. III   = _____

42. V   = _____

43. IX   = _____

44. VII   = _____

45. XI   = _____

46. XIV = _____

47. XVI = _____

48. XII   = _____

49. XVII = _____

50. XIII = _____

To increase your abilities to use either system, convert the following Arabic numbers or Roman numerals.

51. 19   = _____

52. XII = _____

53. 7   = _____

54. IX   = _____

55. IV   = _____

56. 11   = _____

57. VIII = _____

58. 16 = _____

59. XX = _____

60. 5   = _____

61. I   = _____

62. 18 = _____

63. VI = _____

64. 2   = _____

65. III = _____

66. 10 = _____

67. XIII = _____

68. 14 = _____

69. XV = _____

70. 17 = _____

■ FRACTIONS

Medication dosages with fractions are occasionally ordered by the physician or used by the pharmaceutical manufacturer on the drug label. A **fraction** is a number that represents part of a whole number and contains three parts:

1. **Numerator**—the number on the top portion of the fraction that represents the number of parts of the whole fraction.
2. **Dividing line**—the line separating the top portion of the fraction from the bottom portion of the fraction.
3. **Denominator**—the number on the bottom portion of the fraction that represents the number of parts into which the whole is divided.

$$\frac{3}{4} = \frac{\text{numerator}}{\text{denominator}}$$

To solve medication dosage calculation problems using dimensional analysis, you must be able to identify the numerator and denominator portion of the problem. You also must be able to multiply and divide numbers, fractions, and decimals.

Multiplying Fractions

The three steps for multiplying fractions are:

1. Multiply the numerators.
2. Multiply the denominators.
3. Reduce the product to the lowest possible fraction.

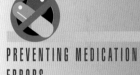

PREVENTING MEDICATION ERRORS

Understanding fractions will assist in preventing **medication errors.** A medication order may include a fraction.
   Example: Administer 1/150 gr of nitroglycerin.

EXAMPLE 1.4

$$\frac{2}{4} \times \frac{1}{8} = \frac{2}{32} = \frac{1}{16}$$

or

$$\frac{2\,(\text{numerator})}{4\,(\text{denominator})} \times \frac{1\,(\text{numerator})}{8\,(\text{denominator})} = \frac{2\;(\text{numerator})}{32\,(\text{denominator})}$$

$$= \frac{1}{16}(\text{reduced to lowest possible fraction})$$

EXAMPLE 1.5

$$\frac{1}{2} \times \frac{2}{4} = \frac{2}{8} = \frac{1}{4}$$

or

$$\frac{1\,(\text{numerator})}{2\,(\text{denominator})} \times \frac{2\,(\text{numerator})}{4\,(\text{denominator})} = \frac{2\,(\text{numerator})}{8\,(\text{denominator})}$$

$$= \frac{1}{4}(\text{reduced to lowest possible fraction})$$

Exercise 1.2   **Multiplying Fractions**
(See pages 23–24 for answers)

To increase your abilities when working with fractions, multiply the following fractions and reduce to the lowest fractional term.

1. $\dfrac{3}{4} \times \dfrac{5}{8} =$

2. $\dfrac{1}{3} \times \dfrac{4}{9} =$

3. $\dfrac{2}{3} \times \dfrac{4}{5} =$

4. $\dfrac{3}{4} \times \dfrac{1}{2} =$

5. $\dfrac{1}{8} \times \dfrac{4}{5} =$

6. $\dfrac{2}{3} \times \dfrac{5}{8} =$

7. $\dfrac{3}{8} \times \dfrac{2}{3} =$

8. $\dfrac{4}{7} \times \dfrac{2}{4} =$

9. $\dfrac{4}{5} \times \dfrac{1}{2} =$

10. $\dfrac{1}{4} \times \dfrac{1}{8} =$

Dividing Fractions

The four steps for dividing fractions are:

1. Invert (turn upside down) the divisor portion of the problem (the second fraction in the problem).
2. Multiply the two numerators.
3. Multiply the two denominators.
4. Reduce answer to lowest term (fraction or whole number).

EXAMPLE 1.6

$$\frac{2}{4} \div \frac{1}{8} = \frac{2}{4} \times \frac{8}{1} = \frac{16}{4} = 4$$

or

$$\frac{2\,(\text{numerator})}{4\,(\text{denominator})} \div \frac{1\,(\text{numerator})}{8\,(\text{denominator})}$$

$$= \frac{2\,(\text{numerator}) \overset{(\text{inverted fraction})}{\times\, 8\,(\text{numerator})} = 16}{4\,(\text{denominator}) \times 1\,(\text{denominator}) = 4}$$

$$= 4\,(\text{answer reduced to lowest term})$$

EXAMPLE 1.7

$$\frac{1}{2} \div \frac{2}{4} = \frac{1}{2} \times \frac{4}{2} = \frac{4}{4} = 1$$

or

$$\frac{1\,(\text{numerator})}{2\,(\text{denominator})} \div \frac{2\,(\text{numerator})}{4\,(\text{denominator})}$$

$$= \frac{1\,(\text{numerator}) \overset{(\text{inverted fraction})}{\times\, 4\,(\text{numerator})} = 4}{2\,(\text{denominator}) \times 2\,(\text{denominator}) = 4}$$

$$= 1\,(\text{answer reduced to lowest term})$$

Exercise 1.3   **Dividing Fractions**
(See page 24 for answers)

To increase your abilities when working with fractions, divide the following fractions and reduce to the lowest fractional term.

1. $\dfrac{3}{4} \div \dfrac{2}{3} =$

2. $\dfrac{1}{9} \div \dfrac{3}{9} =$

3. $\dfrac{2}{3} \div \dfrac{1}{6} =$

4. $\dfrac{1}{5} \div \dfrac{4}{5} =$

5. $\dfrac{3}{6} \div \dfrac{4}{8} =$

6. $\dfrac{5}{8} \div \dfrac{5}{8} =$

7. $\dfrac{1}{8} \div \dfrac{2}{3} =$

8. $\dfrac{1}{5} \div \dfrac{1}{2} =$

9. $\dfrac{1}{4} \div \dfrac{1}{2} =$

10. $\dfrac{1}{6} \div \dfrac{1}{3} =$

■ DECIMALS

Medication orders are often written using decimals, and pharmaceutical manufacturers may use decimals when labeling medications. Therefore, you must understand the learning principles involving decimals and be able to multiply and divide decimals.

- A decimal point is preceded by a zero if not preceded by a number to decrease the chance of an error if the decimal point is missed.

EXAMPLE 1.8

0.25

- A decimal point may be preceded by a number and followed by a number.

EXAMPLE 1.9

1.25

- Numbers to the left of the decimal point are *units, tens, hundreds, thousands,* and *ten-thousands.*
- Numbers to the right of the decimal point are *tenths, hundredths, thousandths,* and *ten-thousandths.*

EXAMPLE 1.10

```
  0.2 = 2 tenths
 0.05 = 5 hundredths
 0.25 = 25 hundredths
 1.25 = 1 unit and 25 hundredths
110.25 = 110 units and 25 hundredths
```

Rounding Decimals

- Decimals may be rounded off. If the number to the right of the decimal is greater than or equal to 5, round up to the next number.
- If the number to the right of the decimal is less than 5, delete the remaining numbers.

EXAMPLE 1.11

```
0.78 = 0.8
0.213 = 0.2
```

Exercise 1.4   **Rounding Decimals**
(See page 24 for answers)

Practice rounding off the following decimals to the tenth.

1. 0.75 =

2. 0.88 =

3. 0.44 =

4. 0.23 =

5. 0.67 =

6. 0.27 =

7. 0.98 =

8. 0.92 =

9. 0.64 =

10. 0.250 =

PREVENTING MEDICATION ERRORS

Understanding the importance of a decimal point will assist in preventing **medication errors.** An improper placement of a decimal point can result in a serious medication error. According to the Institute for Safe Medication Practices (ISMP):

Trailing zeros should not be used with whole numbers.

Example: Administer 1 mg of Xanax.

If a decimal point and a zero are placed after the number (1.0 mg), the order could be misread as Administer 10 mg of Xanax.

Leading zeros should ***always*** *precede a decimal point when the dosage is not a whole number.*

Example: Administer 0.125 mg of Lanoxin.

If a zero is not placed in front of the decimal point the order could be misread as Administer 125 mg of Lanoxin.

Multiplying Decimals

When multiplying with decimals, the principles of multiplication still apply. The numbers are multiplied in columns, but the number of decimal points are counted and placed in the answer, counting places from right to left.

EXAMPLE 1.12

$$
\begin{array}{r}
2.3 \text{ (1 decimal point)} \\
\times\, 1.5 \text{ (1 decimal point)} \\
\hline
115 \\
230 \\
\hline
3.45
\end{array}
$$

Exercise 1.5 | **Multiplying Decimals**
(See pages 24–25 for answers)

Practice multiplying the following decimals.

1. $\begin{array}{r} 2.5 \\ \times\, 4.6 \\ \hline \end{array}$

2. $\begin{array}{r} 1.45 \\ \times\, 0.25 \\ \hline \end{array}$

3. $\begin{array}{r} 3.9 \\ \times\, 0.8 \\ \hline \end{array}$

4. $\begin{array}{r} 2.56 \\ \times\, 0.45 \\ \hline \end{array}$

5. $\begin{array}{r} 10.65 \\ \times\, 0.05 \\ \hline \end{array}$

6. $\begin{array}{r} 1.98 \\ \times\, 3.10 \\ \hline \end{array}$

7. $\begin{array}{r} 2.75 \\ \times\, 5.0 \\ \hline \end{array}$

8. $\begin{array}{r} 5.0 \\ \times\, 0.45 \\ \hline \end{array}$

9. $\begin{array}{r} 7.50 \\ \times\, 0.25 \\ \hline \end{array}$

10. $\begin{array}{r} 2.5 \\ \times\, 0.01 \\ \hline \end{array}$

Dividing Decimals

When dividing with decimals, the principles of division still apply, except that the dividing number is changed to a whole number by moving the decimal point to the right. The number being divided also changes by accepting the same number of decimal point moves.

EXAMPLE 1.13

$0.5 \overline{)0.75}$

STEP 1 Move decimal point one place to the right.

STEP 2

$$
\begin{array}{r}
1.5 \\
5\overline{)7.5} \\
\underline{5} \\
25 \\
\underline{25} \\
0
\end{array}
$$

▶ ▶ ▶ *1.5*

Exercise 1.6 Dividing Decimals
(See pages 25–26 for answers)

Practice dividing the following decimals and rounding the answers to the tenth.

1. $3.4 \overline{)9.6}$

2. $0.25 \overline{)12.50}$

3. $0.56 \overline{)18.65}$

4. $0.3 \overline{)0.192}$

5. $0.4 \overline{)12.43}$

6. $0.5 \overline{)12.50}$

7. $0.125 \overline{)0.25}$

8. $0.08 \overline{)0.085}$

9. $1.5 \overline{)22.5}$

10. $5.5 \overline{)16.5}$

■ CONVERTING FRACTIONS TO DECIMALS

When problem solving with dimensional analysis, medication dosage calculation problems may frequently contain both fractions and decimals. Some of you may have fraction phobia and prefer to convert fractions to decimals when solving problems. To convert a fraction to a decimal, divide the numerator portion of the fraction by the denominator portion of the fraction.

When dividing fractions, remember to add a decimal point and a zero if the numerator cannot be divided by the denominator.

EXAMPLE 1.14

$$\frac{1}{2} \text{ or } \frac{1 \text{ (numerator)}}{2 \text{ (denominator)}} = 2\overline{)1.0} \begin{array}{c} 0.5 = 0.5 \\ \underline{1\ 0} \end{array}$$

EXAMPLE 1.15

$$\frac{3}{4} \text{ or } \frac{3 \text{ (numerator)}}{4 \text{ (denominator)}} = 4\overline{)3.00} \begin{array}{c} 0.75 = 0.75 \\ \underline{2\ 8} \\ 20 \\ \underline{20} \end{array}$$

Exercise 1.7   Converting Fractions to Decimals
(See pages 27–28 for answers)

To decrease fraction phobia, practice converting the following fractions to decimals. Remember to follow the rules of rounding.

1. $\dfrac{1}{8} =$

2. $\dfrac{1}{4} =$

3. $\dfrac{2}{5} =$

4. $\dfrac{3}{5} =$

5. $\dfrac{2}{3} =$

6. $\dfrac{6}{8} =$

PREVENTING MEDICATION ERRORS

Understanding the importance of converting fractions to decimals will assist in preventing **medication errors.** Many medication errors occur because of a simple arithmetic error with dividing. Every nurse should have a calculator to recheck answers for accuracy. If a recheck results in a different answer, the next recheck should include consulting with another nurse or pharmacist.

7. $\dfrac{3}{8} =$

8. $\dfrac{1}{3} =$

9. $\dfrac{3}{6} =$

10. $\dfrac{2}{10} =$

Summary

This chapter has reviewed basic arithmetic that will assist you to successfully implement dimensional analysis as a problem-solving method for medication dosage calculations. To assess your understanding and retention, complete the following practice problems.

Practice Problems for Chapter 1	**Arithmetic Review** (See pages 28–29 for answers)

Change the following Arabic numbers to Roman numerals.

1. 2 =

2. 4 =

3. 5 =

4. 14 =

5. 19 =

Change the following Roman numerals to Arabic numbers.

6. VI   =

7. IX   =

8. XII   =

9. XVII =

10. XIX =

Multiply the following fractions and reduce the answer to the lowest fractional term.

11. $\dfrac{3}{4} \times \dfrac{2}{5} =$

12. $\dfrac{2}{3} \times \dfrac{5}{8} =$

13. $\dfrac{1}{2} \times \dfrac{2}{3} =$

14. $\dfrac{7}{8} \times \dfrac{1}{3} =$

15. $\dfrac{4}{5} \times \dfrac{2}{7} =$

Divide the following fractions and reduce the answer to the lowest fractional term.

16. $\dfrac{1}{2} \div \dfrac{3}{4} =$

17. $\dfrac{1}{3} \div \dfrac{7}{8} =$

18. $\dfrac{1}{5} \div \dfrac{1}{2} =$

19. $\dfrac{4}{8} \div \dfrac{2}{3} =$

20. $\dfrac{1}{3} \div \dfrac{2}{3} =$

Multiply the following decimals.

21. $\begin{array}{r} 6.45 \\ \times\, 1.36 \\ \hline \end{array}$

22. $\begin{array}{r} 3.14 \\ \times\, 2.20 \\ \hline \end{array}$

23. $\begin{array}{r} 16.286 \\ \times\, 0.125 \\ \hline \end{array}$

24. $\begin{array}{r} 1.2 \\ \times\, 0.5 \\ \hline \end{array}$

25. $\begin{array}{r} 7.68 \\ \times\, 0.05 \\ \hline \end{array}$

Divide the following decimals.

26. $0.5\overline{)1.25}$

27. $0.20\overline{)40.80}$

28. $0.125\overline{)0.25}$

29. $0.75\overline{)0.125}$

30. $0.5\overline{)7.30}$

(Practice Problems continue on page 20)

Convert the following fractions to decimals and round to the tenth.

31. $\dfrac{1}{2} =$

32. $\dfrac{1}{3} =$

33. $\dfrac{3}{4} =$

34. $\dfrac{2}{3} =$

35. $\dfrac{1}{8} =$

Chapter 1 Post-Test: Arithmetic Review

Name _____ **Date** _____

Converting Between Arabic Numbers and Roman Numerals

1. 4 = _____

2. IX = _____

3. 16 = _____

4. XXV = _____

Multiplying and Dividing Fractions

5. $\dfrac{1}{8} \times \dfrac{1}{8} =$ _____

6. $\dfrac{2}{4} \times \dfrac{1}{2} =$ _____

7. $\dfrac{5}{6} \times \dfrac{3}{4} =$ _____

8. $\dfrac{1}{6} \div \dfrac{1}{3} =$ _____

9. $\dfrac{3}{4} \div \dfrac{7}{8} =$ _____

10. $\dfrac{1}{150} \div \dfrac{1}{2} =$ _____

Converting Fractions to Decimals

11. $\dfrac{1}{2} =$ _____

12. $\dfrac{3}{4} =$ _____

13. $\dfrac{7}{8} =$ _____

14. $\dfrac{2}{3} =$ _____

Multiplying and Dividing Decimals

15. $0.25 \times 1.25 =$ _____

16. $0.125 \div 0.25 =$ _____

17. $0.55 \times 0.75 =$ _____

18. $1.5 \times 0.25 =$ _____

19. $0.125 \div 0.5 =$ _____

20. $0.525 \div 0.3 =$ _____

ANSWER KEY FOR CHAPTER 1: ARITHMETIC REVIEW

Exercise 1.1 **Arabic Numbers and Roman Numerals**

1. 1 = I
2. 1 + 1 = II
3. 1 + 1 + 1 = III
4. 5 − 1 = IV
5. 5 = V
6. 5 + 1 = VI
7. 5 + 1 + 1 = VII
8. 5 + 1 + 1 + 1 = VIII
9. 10 − 1 = IX
10. 10 = X
11. 10 + 1 = XI
12. 10 + 1 + 1 = XII
13. 10 + 1 + 1 + 1 = XIII
14. 10 + 5 − 1 = XIV
15. 10 + 5 = XV
16. 10 + 5 + 1 = XVI
17. 10 + 5 + 1 + 1 = XVII
18. 10 + 5 + 1 + 1 + 1 = XVIII
19. 10 + 10 − 1 = XIX
20. 10 + 10 = XX
21. 50 − 10 + 1 + 1 + 1 = XLIII
22. 10 + 10 + 5 − 1 = XXIV
23. 50 + 5 = LV
24. 10 + 10 + 10 + 1 + 1 = XXXII
25. 100 + 1 + 1 = CII
26. 100 + 50 = CL
27. 50 + 10 + 10 + 5 = LXXV
28. 100 − 10 + 1 + 1 = XCII
29. 50 + 10 + 5 − 1 = LXIV
30. 50 + 10 + 10 − 1 = LXIX
31. II = (1 + 1) = 2
32. IV = (5 − 1) = 4
33. VI = (5 + 1) = 6
34. X = (10) = 10
35. VIII = (5 + 1 + 1 + 1) = 8
36. XIX = (10 − 1 + 10) = 19
37. XX = (10 + 10) = 20
38. XVIII = (10 + 5 + 1 + 1 + 1) = 18
39. I = (1) = 1
40. XV = (10 + 5) = 15
41. III = (1 + 1 + 1) = 3
42. V = (5) = 5
43. IX = (10 − 1) = 9
44. VII = (5 + 1 + 1) = 7
45. XI = (10 + 1) = 11
46. XIV = (10 + 5 − 1) = 14
47. XVI = (10 + 5 + 1) = 16
48. XII = (10 + 1 + 1) = 12
49. XVII = (10 + 5 + 1 + 1) = 17
50. XIII = (10 + 1 + 1 + 1) = 13
51. 19 = XIX
52. XII = 12
53. 7 = VII
54. IX = 9
55. IV = 4
56. 11 = XI
57. VIII = 8
58. 16 = XVI
59. XX = 20
60. 5 = V
61. I = 1
62. 18 = XVIII
63. VI = 6
64. 2 = II
65. III = 3
66. 10 = X
67. XIII = 13
68. 14 = XIV
69. XV = 15
70. 17 = XVII

Exercise 1.2 **Multiplying Fractions**

1. $\dfrac{3}{4} \times \dfrac{5}{8} = \dfrac{3 \times 5 = 15}{4 \times 8 = 32} = \dfrac{15}{32}$

2. $\dfrac{1}{3} \times \dfrac{4}{9} = \dfrac{1 \times 4 = 4}{3 \times 9 = 27} = \dfrac{4}{27}$

3. $\dfrac{2}{3} \times \dfrac{4}{5} = \dfrac{2 \times 4 = 8}{3 \times 5 = 15} = \dfrac{8}{15}$

4. $\dfrac{3}{4} \times \dfrac{1}{2} = \dfrac{3 \times 1 = 3}{4 \times 2 = 8} = \dfrac{3}{8}$

5. $\dfrac{1}{8} \times \dfrac{4}{5} = \dfrac{1 \times 4 = 4(4) = 1}{8 \times 5 = 40(4) = 10} = \dfrac{1}{10}$

6. $\dfrac{2}{3} \times \dfrac{5}{8} = \dfrac{2 \times 5 = 10(2) = 5}{3 \times 8 = 24(2) = 12} = \dfrac{5}{12}$

7. $\dfrac{3}{8} \times \dfrac{2}{3} = \dfrac{3 \times 2 = 6(6) = 1}{8 \times 3 = 24(6) = 4} = \dfrac{1}{4}$

8. $\dfrac{4}{7} \times \dfrac{2}{4} = \dfrac{4 \times 2 = 8(4) = 2}{7 \times 4 = 28(4) = 7} = \dfrac{2}{7}$

9. $\frac{4}{5} \times \frac{1}{2} = \frac{4 \times 1 = 4(2) = 2}{5 \times 2 = 10(2) = 5} = \frac{2}{5}$

10. $\frac{1}{4} \times \frac{1}{8} = \frac{1 \times 1 = 1}{4 \times 8 = 32} = \frac{1}{32}$

Exercise 1.3 **Dividing Fractions**

1. $\frac{3}{4} \div \frac{2}{3} = \frac{3}{4} \times \frac{3}{2}$ or $\frac{3 \times 3 = 9}{4 \times 2 = 8} = 8\overline{)9}^{1\frac{1}{8}} = 1\frac{1}{8}$
$\frac{8}{1}$

2. $\frac{1}{9} \div \frac{3}{9} = \frac{1}{9} \times \frac{9}{3}$ or $\frac{1 \times 9 = 9(9) = 1}{9 \times 3 = 27(9) = 3} = \frac{1}{3}$

3. $\frac{2}{3} \div \frac{1}{6} = \frac{2}{3} \times \frac{6}{1}$ or $\frac{2 \times 6 = 12}{3 \times 1 = 3} = 3\overline{)12}^{4} = 4$
$\underline{12}$

4. $\frac{1}{5} \div \frac{4}{5} = \frac{1}{5} \times \frac{5}{4}$ or $\frac{1 \times 5 = 5(5) = 1}{5 \times 4 = 20(5) = 4} = \frac{1}{4}$

5. $\frac{3}{6} \div \frac{4}{8} = \frac{3}{6} \times \frac{8}{4}$ or $\frac{3 \times 8 = 24}{6 \times 4 = 24} = 24\overline{)24}^{1} = 1$

6. $\frac{5}{8} \div \frac{5}{8} = \frac{5}{8} \times \frac{8}{5}$ or $\frac{5 \times 8 = 40}{8 \times 5 = 40} = 40\overline{)40}^{1} = 1$

7. $\frac{1}{8} \div \frac{2}{3} = \frac{1}{8} \times \frac{3}{2}$ or $\frac{1 \times 3 = 3}{8 \times 2 = 16} = \frac{3}{16}$

8. $\frac{1}{5} \div \frac{1}{2} = \frac{1}{5} \times \frac{2}{1}$ or $\frac{1 \times 2 = 2}{5 \times 1 = 5} = \frac{2}{5}$

9. $\frac{1}{4} \div \frac{1}{2} = \frac{1 \times 2 = 2(2) = 1}{4 \times 1 = 4(2) = 2} = \frac{1}{2}$

10. $\frac{1}{6} \div \frac{1}{3} = \frac{1 \times 3 = 3(3) = 1}{6 \times 1 = 6(3) = 2} = \frac{1}{2}$

Exercise 1.4 **Rounding Decimals**

1. 0.75 = 0.8
2. 0.88 = 0.9
3. 0.44 = 0.4
4. 0.23 = 0.2
5. 0.67 = 0.7
6. 0.27 = 0.3
7. 0.98 = 1
8. 0.92 = 0.9
9. 0.64 = 0.6
10. 0.250 = 0.3

Exercise 1.5 **Multiplying Decimals**

1.   2.5 (1 decimal point)
   $\times$ 4.6 (1 decimal point)
   150
   $\underline{1000}$
   1150
   11.50 (2 decimal points from the right to left)

2.   1.45 (2 decimal points)
   $\times$ 0.25 (2 decimal points)
   725
   2900
   $\underline{0000}$
   3625
   0.3625 (4 decimal points from the right to left)

3.   3.9 (1 decimal point)
   $\times$ 0.8 (1 decimal point)
   312
   $\underline{000}$
   312
   3.12 (2 decimal points from the right to left)

4.   2.56 (2 decimal points)
   $\times$ 0.45 (2 decimal points)
   1280
   10240
   $\underline{00000}$
   11520
   1.1520 (4 decimal points from the right to left)

5.   10.65 (2 decimal points)
   $\times$ 0.05 (2 decimal points)
   5325
   $\underline{0000}$
   5325
   0.5325 (4 decimal points from the right to left)

6.   1.98 (2 decimal points)
    × 3.10 (2 decimal points)
        000
       1980
     59400
    61380
    6.1380 (4 decimal points from the right to left)

7.   2.75 (2 decimal points)
    × 5.0 (1 decimal point)
        000
    13750
    13750
    13.750 (3 decimal points from the right to left)

8.   5.0 (1 decimal point)
    × 0.45 (2 decimal points)
      250
    2000
    0000
    2250
    2.250 (3 decimal points from the right to left)

9.   7.50 (2 decimal points)
    × 0.25 (2 decimal points)
     3750
   15000
   00000
   18750
   1.8750 (4 decimal points from the right to left)

10.   2.5 (1 decimal point)
    × 0.01 (2 decimal points)
      25
    000
    0000
    0025
    0.025 (3 decimal points from the right to left)

Exercise 1.6 Dividing Decimals

1. $3.4\overline{)9.6}$

(Move decimal points one place to the right)

Answer: 2.82 = 2.8

$$
\begin{array}{r}
2.82 \\
34\overline{)96.00} \\
\underline{68} \\
28\ 0 \\
\underline{27\ 2} \\
80 \\
\underline{68} \\
12
\end{array}
$$

2. $0.25\overline{)12.50}$

(Move decimal points two places to the right)

Answer: 50. = 50

$$
\begin{array}{r}
50. \\
25\overline{)1250.} \\
\underline{125} \\
00
\end{array}
$$

3. $0.56\overline{)18.65}$

(Move decimal points two places to the right)

Answer: 33.30 = 33.3

$$
\begin{array}{r}
33.30 \\
56\overline{)1865.00} \\
\underline{168} \\
185 \\
\underline{168} \\
170 \\
\underline{168} \\
20
\end{array}
$$

4. $0.3\overline{)0.192}$

(Move decimal points one place to the right)

Answer: 0.64 = 0.6

$$
\begin{array}{r}
0.64 \\
3\overline{)01.92} \\
\underline{18} \\
12 \\
\underline{12} \\
0
\end{array}
$$

5. $0.4\overline{)12.43}$

(Move decimal points one place to the right)

Answer: $31.075 = 31.1$

$$
\begin{array}{r}
31.075 \\
4\overline{)124.300} \\
\underline{12} \\
04 \\
\underline{4} \\
030 \\
\underline{28} \\
20 \\
\underline{20} \\
0
\end{array}
$$

6. $0.5\overline{)12.50}$

(Move decimal points one place to the right)

Answer: $25.0 = 25$

$$
\begin{array}{r}
25.0 \\
5\overline{)125.0} \\
\underline{10} \\
25 \\
\underline{25} \\
0
\end{array}
$$

7. $0.125\overline{)0.25}$

(Move decimal points three places to the right)

Answer: $2. = 2$

$$
\begin{array}{r}
2 \\
125\overline{)250} \\
\underline{250} \\
0
\end{array}
$$

8. $0.08\overline{)0.085}$

(Move decimal points two places to the right)

Answer: $1.0625 = 1.1$

$$
\begin{array}{r}
1.0625 \\
8\overline{)8.5000} \\
\underline{8} \\
50 \\
\underline{48} \\
20 \\
\underline{16} \\
40 \\
\underline{40} \\
0
\end{array}
$$

9. $1.5\overline{)22.5}$

(Move decimal points one place to the right)

Answer: $15. = 15$

$$
\begin{array}{r}
15. \\
15.\overline{)225.} \\
\underline{15} \\
75 \\
\underline{75}
\end{array}
$$

10. $5.5\overline{)16.5}$

(Move decimal points one place to the right)

Answer: $3. = 3$

$$
\begin{array}{r}
3. \\
55.\overline{)165.} \\
\underline{165}
\end{array}
$$

**Exercise 1.7 Converting Fractions
to Decimals**

1. $\dfrac{1}{8} = 0.125 = 0.13 = 0.1$

   Answer: 0.1

   $$\begin{array}{r} 0.125 \\ 8\overline{)1.000} \\ \underline{8} \\ 20 \\ \underline{16} \\ 40 \\ \underline{40} \\ 0 \end{array}$$

2. $\dfrac{1}{4} = 0.25 = 0.3$

   Answer: 0.3

   $$\begin{array}{r} .25 \\ 4\overline{)1.00} \\ \underline{8} \\ 20 \\ \underline{20} \\ 0 \end{array}$$

3. $\dfrac{2}{5} = 0.4$

   Answer: 0.4

   $$\begin{array}{r} 0.4 \\ 5\overline{)2.0} \\ \underline{20} \\ 0 \end{array}$$

4. $\dfrac{3}{5} = 0.6$

   Answer: 0.6

   $$\begin{array}{r} 0.6 \\ 5\overline{)3.0} \\ \underline{30} \\ 0 \end{array}$$

5. $\dfrac{2}{3} = 0.66 = 0.7$

   Answer: 0.7

   $$\begin{array}{r} 0.66 \\ 3\overline{)2.00} \\ \underline{1\,8} \\ 20 \\ \underline{18} \\ 2 \end{array}$$

6. $\dfrac{6}{8} = 0.75 = 0.8$

   Answer: 0.8

   $$\begin{array}{r} 0.75 \\ 8\overline{)6.00} \\ \underline{56} \\ 40 \\ \underline{40} \\ 0 \end{array}$$

7. $\dfrac{3}{8} = 0.375 = 0.38 = 0.4$

   Answer: 0.4

   $$\begin{array}{r} 0.375 \\ 8\overline{)3.00} \\ \underline{2\,4} \\ 60 \\ \underline{56} \\ 40 \\ \underline{40} \\ 0 \end{array}$$

8. $\dfrac{1}{3} = 0.33 = 0.3$

   Answer: 0.3

   $$\begin{array}{r} 0.33 \\ 3\overline{)1.00} \\ \underline{9} \\ 10 \\ \underline{9} \\ 1 \end{array}$$

9. $\dfrac{3}{6} = 0.5$

Answer: 0.5

$$6\overline{)3.0}^{\;0.5}$$
$$\underline{30}$$
$$0$$

10. $\dfrac{2}{10} = 0.2$

Answer: 0.2

$$10\overline{)2.0}^{\;0.2}$$
$$\underline{20}$$
$$0$$

Practice Problems

1. II
2. IV
3. V
4. XIV
5. XIX
6. 6
7. 9
8. 12
9. 17
10. 19

11. $\dfrac{3 \times 2 = 6\,(2) = 3}{4 \times 5 = 20\,(2) = 10} = \dfrac{3}{10}$

12. $\dfrac{2 \times 5 = 10\,(2) = 5}{3 \times 8 = 24\,(2) = 12} = \dfrac{5}{12}$

13. $\dfrac{1 \times 2 = 2\,(2) = 1}{2 \times 3 = 6\,(2) = 3} = \dfrac{1}{3}$

14. $\dfrac{7 \times 1 = 7}{8 \times 3 = 24} = \dfrac{7}{24}$

15. $\dfrac{4 \times 2 = 8}{5 \times 7 = 35} = \dfrac{8}{35}$

16. $\dfrac{1}{2} \div \dfrac{3}{4} = \dfrac{1 \times 4 = 4\,(2) = 2}{2 \times 3 = 6\,(2) = 3} = \dfrac{2}{3}$

17. $\dfrac{1}{3} \div \dfrac{7}{8} = \dfrac{1 \times 8 = 8}{3 \times 7 = 21} = \dfrac{8}{21}$

18. $\dfrac{1}{5} \div \dfrac{1}{2} = \dfrac{1 \times 2 = 2}{5 \times 1 = 5} = \dfrac{2}{5}$

19. $\dfrac{4}{8} \div \dfrac{2}{3} = \dfrac{4 \times 3 = 12\,(4) = 3}{8 \times 2 = 16\,(4) = 4} = \dfrac{3}{4}$

20. $\dfrac{1}{3} \div \dfrac{2}{3} = \dfrac{1 \times 3 = 3\,(3) = 1}{3 \times 2 = 6\,(3) = 2} = \dfrac{1}{2}$

21.   6.45 (2 decimal points)
$\times \underline{1.36}$ (2 decimal points)
   3870
19350
$\underline{64500}$
87720
8.7720 (4 decimal points from right to left)

22.   3.14 (2 decimal points)
$\times \underline{\;2.20}$ (2 decimal points)
    000
   6280
$\underline{62800}$
69080
6.9080 (4 decimal points from right to left)

23.   16.286 (3 decimal points)
$\times \underline{0.125}$ (3 decimal points)
   81430
  325720
$\underline{1628600}$
2035750
2.035750 (6 decimal points from right to le

24.   1.2 (1 decimal point)
$\times \underline{0.5}$ (1 decimal point)
   60
$\underline{000}$
060
0.60 (2 decimal points from right to left)

25.   7.68 (2 decimal points)
$\times \underline{0.05}$ (2 decimal points)
   3840
  0000
$\underline{00000}$
03840
0.3840 (4 decimal points from right to left)

26. $0.5\overline{)1.25}$

(Move decimal points one place to the right)

Answer: 2.5

$$
\begin{array}{r}
2.5 \\
5\overline{)12.5} \\
\underline{10} \\
25 \\
\underline{25} \\
0
\end{array}
$$

27. $0.20\overline{)40.80}$

(Move decimal points two places to the right)

Answer: 204. = 204

$$
\begin{array}{r}
204 \\
20\overline{)4080} \\
\underline{40} \\
080 \\
\underline{80} \\
0
\end{array}
$$

28. $0.125\overline{)0.25}$

(Move decimal points three places to the right)

Answer: 2. = 2

$$
\begin{array}{r}
2 \\
125\overline{)250} \\
\underline{250} \\
0
\end{array}
$$

29. $0.75\overline{)0.125}$

(Move decimal points two places to the right)

Answer: 0.166 = 0.17 = 0.2

$$
\begin{array}{r}
0.166 \\
75\overline{)12.500} \\
\underline{75} \\
500 \\
\underline{450} \\
50
\end{array}
$$

30. $0.5\overline{)7.30}$

(Move decimal point one place to the right)

Answer: 14.6

$$
\begin{array}{r}
14.6 \\
5\overline{)73.0} \\
\underline{5} \\
23 \\
\underline{20} \\
30 \\
\underline{30} \\
0
\end{array}
$$

31. 0.5
32. 0.33 = 0.3
33. 0.75 = 0.8
34. 0.66 = 0.7
35. 0.125 = 0.13 = 0.1

CHAPTER **2**

Systems of Measurement and Common Equivalents

Objectives

After completing this chapter, you will successfully be able to:

1. **Identify measurements included in the metric, apothecaries', and household systems.**
2. **Understand abbreviations used in the metric, apothecaries', and household systems.**
3. **Calculate intake and output necessary for accurate recording in a medical record.**
4. **Differentiate between Fahrenheit and Celsius thermometers used for monitoring temperature.**
5. **Differentiate between standard time and military time necessary for accurate recording in a medical record.**

Outline

Medication calculation need not be difficult if you have a problem-solving method that is easy to understand and implement. In addition, you need to understand common equivalents and units of measurement to visualize all parts of a medication dosage calculation problem. Understanding common equivalents and units of measurement will assist you in preventing **medication errors** related to incorrect dosage.

This chapter will help you to understand the measurement systems used for medication administration. This knowledge is necessary to accurately implement the problem-solving method of dimensional analysis.

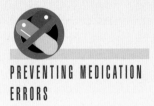

PREVENTING MEDICATION ERRORS

■ SYSTEMS OF MEASUREMENT

Three systems of measurement are used for medication dosage administration: the metric system, the apothecaries' system, and the household system. To be able to accurately administer medication, you must understand all three of these systems.

The Metric System

The **metric system** is a decimal system of weights and measures based on units of ten in which gram, meter, and liter are the basic units of measurement. However, gram and liter are the only measurements from the metric system that are used in medication administration. The meter is a unit of distance, the gram (abbreviated g or gm) is a unit of weight, and the liter (abbreviated L) is a unit of volume.

The most frequently used metric units of *weight* and their equivalents are summarized in Box 2.1.

Another way to understand the metric units of weight and their equivalents is to visualize the relationship between the measurements and equivalents displayed in Figure 2.1.

The most frequently used metric units for *volume* and their equivalents are summarized in Box 2.2.

■ **BOX 2.1**	**Metric System Units of Weight and Equivalents**
	1 kilogram (kg) 1 gram (g) 1 milligram (mg) 1 microgram (mcg) 1 kg = 1000 g 1 g = 1000 mg 1 mg = 1000 mcg

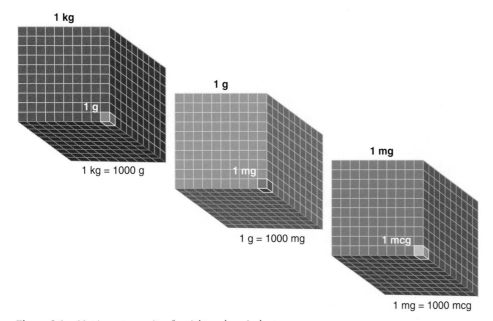

Figure 2.1.   Metric system units of weight and equivalents.

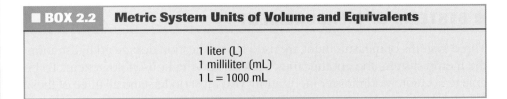

■ BOX 2.2	Metric System Units of Volume and Equivalents

1 liter (L)
1 milliliter (mL)
1 L = 1000 mL

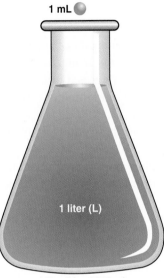

1 mL

1 liter (L)

1 liter (L) = 1000 mL

Figure 2.2.   Metric system units of volume and equivalents.

Another way to understand the metric units of volume and their equivalents is to visualize the relationship between the measurements and equivalents displayed in Figure 2.2.

The Apothecaries' System

The **apothecaries' system** is a system of measuring and weighing drugs and solutions in which fractions are used to identify parts of the unit of measure. The basic units of measurement in the apothecaries' system include weights and liquid volume. Although the apothecaries' system may be replaced by the metric system, it is still necessary to understand it because some physicians continue to order medications using this system, and they also may include Roman numerals in the medication order.

The most frequently used measurements and equivalents within the apothecaries' system's units of *weight* are summarized in Box 2.3, and the most frequently used measurements and equivalents within the apothecaries' system's units of *volume* are summarized in Box 2.4. Figure 2.3 can help you visualize the equivalents for weight and volume.

The Household System

The use of household measurements is considered inaccurate because of the varying sizes of cups, glasses, and eating utensils, and this system generally has been replaced with the metric system. However, as patient care moves away from hospitals, which use the metric system, and into the community, it is once again necessary for the nurse to have an understanding of the household measurement system to be able to use and teach it to clients and families.

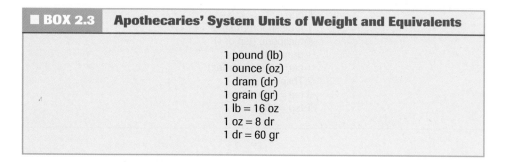

■ BOX 2.3   **Apothecaries' System Units of Weight and Equivalents**

1 pound (lb)
1 ounce (oz)
1 dram (dr)
1 grain (gr)
1 lb = 16 oz
1 oz = 8 dr
1 dr = 60 gr

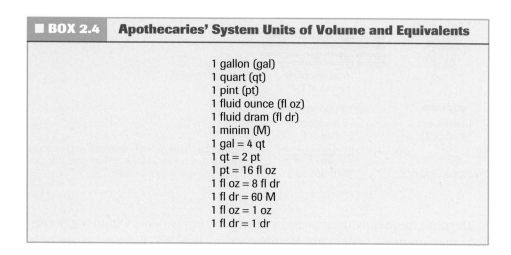

■ BOX 2.4   **Apothecaries' System Units of Volume and Equivalents**

1 gallon (gal)
1 quart (qt)
1 pint (pt)
1 fluid ounce (fl oz)
1 fluid dram (fl dr)
1 minim (M)
1 gal = 4 qt
1 qt = 2 pt
1 pt = 16 fl oz
1 fl oz = 8 fl dr
1 fl dr = 60 M
1 fl oz = 1 oz
1 fl dr = 1 dr

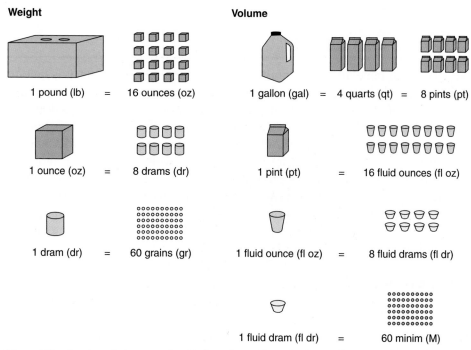

Weight

1 pound (lb) = 16 ounces (oz)

1 ounce (oz) = 8 drams (dr)

1 dram (dr) = 60 grains (gr)

Volume

1 gallon (gal) = 4 quarts (qt) = 8 pints (pt)

1 pint (pt) = 16 fluid ounces (fl oz)

1 fluid ounce (fl oz) = 8 fluid drams (fl dr)

1 fluid dram (fl dr) = 60 minim (M)

Figure 2.3. Apothecaries' system of equivalents for weight and volume. Please note that the figures are not shown to scale.

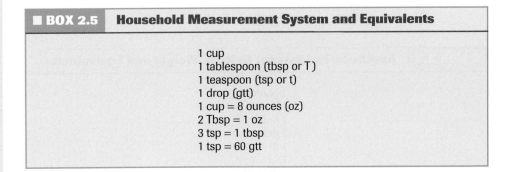

■ BOX 2.5	Household Measurement System and Equivalents

1 cup
1 tablespoon (tbsp or T)
1 teaspoon (tsp or t)
1 drop (gtt)
1 cup = 8 ounces (oz)
2 Tbsp = 1 oz
3 tsp = 1 tbsp
1 tsp = 60 gtt

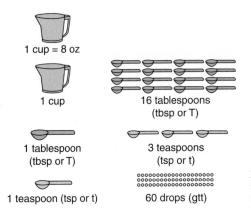

1 cup = 8 oz

1 cup   16 tablespoons (tbsp or T)

1 tablespoon (tbsp or T)   3 teaspoons (tsp or t)

1 teaspoon (tsp or t)   60 drops (gtt)

Figure 2.4. Household measurement system and equivalents for volume. Please note that the figures are not shown to scale.

The most frequently used measurements and equivalents within the household measurement system are summarized in Box 2.5. Figure 2.4 can help you visualize the equivalents.

■ INTAKE AND OUTPUT

Now that you have an understanding of the common equivalents, it is time to utilize that knowledge by calculating the intake from a patient's meal tray. Monitoring the intake of patients is an extremely important nursing function as it provides information regarding fluid retention or fluid loss. If a patient is retaining fluid, the physician or nurse practitioner may need to order a medication to increase the excretion of the fluid as well as limit fluid intake to prevent fluid overload. If a patient is losing fluid, the physician or nurse practitioner may need to increase fluid intake to prevent dehydration. Regardless of the fluid problem, it is the nurse who monitors fluid intake and output to report to the physician or nurse practitioner. Figure 2.5 provides an example of a typical Intake and Output Record.

Temperature

Clients and families are required to monitor temperature changes associated with various medical conditions. Two thermometers may be used for monitoring temperature: a Fahrenheit thermometer or a Celsius thermometer. The nurse must be able to explain both of these systems of measurement when discharging clients and families.

The most frequently used measurements for Celsius and Fahrenheit are summarized in Figure 2.6.

Intake and Output Record				
Name:				
Date:				
INTAKE		**OUTPUT**		
	Oral		Voided	Catheter
Breakfast		**Day Shift**		
		0700		
		0800		
AM Snack		0900		
		1000		
		1100		
Lunch		1200		
		1300		
PM Snack		1400		
		Shift Total		
Dinner		**Evening Shift**		
		1500		
		1600		
		1700		
		1800		
Evening Snack		1900		
		2000		
		2100		
		2200		
		Shift Total		
Common Intake Equivalents:		**Night Shift**		
Large Glass = 240 mL		2300		
Water Glass = 180 mL		2400		
Juice Glass = 120 mL				
Coffee Cup = 240 mL		0100		
Styrofoam Cup = 180 mL		0200		
Large Milk Carton = 240 mL		0300		
Small Milk Carton = 120 mL		0400		
Jello Cup = 120 mL		0500		
Large Soup Bowl = 200 mL		0500		
Small Soup Bowl = 100 mL		0600		
Hot Cereal = 100 mL		**Shift Total**		
Ice Cream = 90 mL				
Popsicle = 80 mL				
Pop Can = 355 mL				
24-Hour Total Intake		**24-Hour Total Output**		

Figure 2.5. Intake and Output Record.

Box 2.6 summarizes a method for converting between Celsius and Fahrenheit or Fahrenheit and Celsius. This easy method requires addition, subtraction, multiplication, or division.

■ TIME

Another conversion that is necessary to learn is the conversion of standard time to military time. Military time has been adopted by all branches of the armed forces, emergency systems, and health care facilities to avoid confusion regarding the AM (morning) and PM (afternoon/evening) administration of medications. When documenting the administration of medications on the medication

Conversion Chart		
Celsius	**to**	**Fahrenheit**
35.0		95.0
35.5		95.9
36.0		96.8
36.5		97.7
37.0		98.6
37.5		99.5
38.0		100.4
38.5		101.3
39.0		102.2
39.5		103.1
40.0		104.0
40.5		104.9
41.0		105.8
41.5		106.7
42.0		107.6

Figure 2.6. Conversion chart for Celsius to Fahrenheit.

administration record (MAR), it is essential that the exact time is noted. Military time uses a 24-hour clock and as the hour hand moves around the clock each hour is clearly identified from 0100 to 1200. After 1200 (noon), the number 12 is added to each number the second time around the clock. Minutes and seconds are recorded the same for standard time and military time but no colon (:) is used to separate the hours and minutes in military time. However, if seconds are to be included in military time then minutes and seconds are separated by a colon (1400:15). Midnight can be referred to as 0000 or 2400 but after midnight the numbers revert to 0100 to 1200. Figure 2.7 displays standard time and military time using a conversion table and Figure 2.8 displays standard time and military time using the face of a clock. Watches are manufactured with standard time and military time visible on the face of a clock to eliminate confusion but learning the conversions is the best method of avoiding errors.

■ COMMON EQUIVALENTS

Sometimes it is necessary to convert from one system to another to accurately administer medication. See Table 2.1 for approximate equivalents for weight and Table 2.2 for approximate equivalents for volume.

■ BOX 2.6   Temperature Conversion Method

To convert from Fahrenheit to Celsius:
$$^{\circ}C = (^{\circ}F - 32) \div 1.8$$

To convert from Celsius to Fahrenheit:
$$^{\circ}F = {}^{\circ}C \times 1.8 + 32$$

$^{\circ}C$ = temperature in degrees Celsius
$^{\circ}F$ = temperature in degrees Fahrenheit

Standard Time	Military Time	Standard Time	Military Time
1:00 am	0100	1:00 pm	12+1 = 1300
1:05 am	0105	1:05 pm	1305
2:00 am	0200	2:00 pm	12+2 = 1400
2:10 am	0210	2:10 pm	1410
3:00 am	0300	3:00 pm	12+3 = 1500
3:15 am	0315	3:15 pm	1515
4:00 am	0400	4:00 pm	12+4 = 1600
4:20 am	0420	4:20 pm	1620
5:00 am	0500	5:00 pm	12+5 = 1700
5:25 am	0525	5:25 pm	1725
6:00 am	0600	6:00 pm	12+6 = 1800
6:30 am	0630	6:30 pm	1830
7:00 am	0700	7:00 pm	12+7 = 1900
7:35 am	0735	7:35 pm	1935
8:00 am	0800	8:00 pm	12+8 = 2000
8:40 am	0840	8:40 pm	2040
9:00 am	0900	9:00 pm	12+9 = 2100
9:45 am	0945	9:45 pm	2145
10:00 am	1000	10:00 pm	12+10 = 2200
10:50 am	1050	10:50 pm	2250
11:00 am	1100	11:00 pm	12+11 = 2300
11:55 am	1155	11:55 pm	2355
12:00 pm (noon)	1200	12:00 am	12+12 = 2400

Figure 2.7. Standard Time and Military Time.

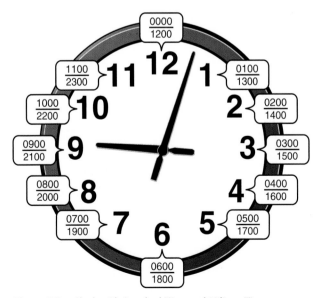

Figure 2.8. Clock with Standard Time and Military Time.

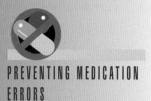

PREVENTING MEDICATION ERRORS

Understanding the three systems of measurement will assist in preventing **medication errors.** Every nurse should have a chart that clearly identifies the conversions between the three systems of measurement to recheck answers for accuracy but it is also the responsibility of the nurse to memorize the equivalents as a chart may not always be available.

■ TABLE 2.1	Approximate Equivalents for Weight
METRIC	**APOTHECARIES'**
1 kg (1000 g)	2.2 lb
1 g (1000 mg)	15 gr
60 mg	1 gr

■ TABLE 2.2	Approximate Equivalents for Volume	
METRIC	**APOTHECARIES'**	**HOUSEHOLD**
4000 mL	1 gal (4 qt)	
1 L (1000 mL)	1 qt (2 pt)	
500 mL	1 pt (16 fl oz)	
240 mL	8 oz	1 cup (1 glass)
30 mL	1 oz (8 dr)	2 tbsp
15 mL	½ oz (4 dr)	1 tbsp (3 tsp)
5 mL	1 dr (60 M)	1 tsp (60 gtt)
1 mL	15 M	15 gtt
	1 M	1 gtt

Summary

This chapter has reviewed the metric, apothecaries', and household systems of measurement. Calculation of intake and output was explained. This chapter also reviewed Fahrenheit and Celsius as well as standard time and military time. To assess your understanding and retention of these systems of measurement, complete the following practice problems.

Practice Problems for Chapter 2 | **Systems of Measurement and Common Equivalents**
(See page 45 for answers)

Write the correct abbreviation symbols for the following measurements from the metric system:

1. kilogram   =   5. liter   =

2. gram   =   6. milliliter =

3. milligram =

4. microgram =

Write the correct abbreviation symbols for the following measurements from the apothecaries' system:

7. pound =   12. quart   =

8. ounce =   13. pint   =

9. dram =   14. fluid ounce =

10. grain =   15. fluid dram =

11. gallon =   16. minim   =

Write the correct abbreviation symbols for the following measurements from the household system:

17. tablespoon =

18. teaspoon   =

19. drop   =

Identify the correct numerical values for the following measurements:

20. 1 kg = _____ lb

21. 1 kg = _____ g

22. 1 g   = _____ mg

23. 1 mg = _____ mcg

24. 1 g   = _____ gr

(Practice Problems continue on page 40)

Calculate the intake for the following meal trays:

25. Breakfast:

Coffee Cup	= 240 mL (drank ½)
Water Glass	= 180 mL (drank ½ with AM medications)
Juice Glass	= 120 mL (drank all)
Hot Cereal	= 100 mL (ate ½)
Total	=

26. Lunch:

Coffee Cup	= 240 mL (drank all)
Small Milk Carton	= 120 mL (drank all)
Large Soup Bowl	= 200 mL (ate ½)
Jello Cup	= 120 mL
Total	=

27. Dinner:

Coffee Cup	= 240 mL (drank ¼)
Large Milk Carton	= 240 mL (drank ½)
Ice Cream	= 90 mL (ate all)
Total	=

Identify the correct numerical values for the following temperatures:

28. 98.6°F = _____ °C

29. 39°C   = _____ °F

30. 104.9°F = _____ °C

31. 36°C   = _____ °F

32. 101.3°F = _____ °C

Convert the following Standard Times to Military Time:

33. 1:00 am   =

34. 5:00 pm   =

35. 3:00 am   =

36. 8:00 pm   =

37. midnight =

Convert the following Military Times to Standard Time:

38. 0230 =

39. 1600 =

40. 0420 =

41. 1200 =

42. 2110 =

Identify the correct numerical values for the following measurements:

43. 1 gr   = ____ mg

44. 1000 mg = ____ g

45. 1000 mL = ____ L   = ____ qt

46. 500 mL = ____ pt

47. 240 mL = ____ oz

48. 30 mL   = ____ oz = ____ tbsp

49. 15 mL   = ____ oz = ____ tsp

50. 5 mL   = ____ tsp

51. 1 mL   = ____ M   = ____ gtt

52. 2 mL   = ____ gtt

53. 30 gtt = ____ M   = ____ mL

54. 4 tbsp = ____ oz = ____ mL

55. 40°C   = ____ °F

56. 1 pt   = ____ fl oz = ____ mL

57. 2 qt   = ____ gal = ____ mL

58. 96.8°F = ____ °C

59. 2000 g = ____ kg = ____ lb

60. gr xv   ____ g   = ____ mg

61. 37.5°C = ____ °F

62. 1 oz   = ____ dr = ____ mL

63. 32 fl oz = ____ pt = ____ mL

64. 39°C   = ____ °F

65. gr xxx = ____ g   = ____ mg

66. 240 mL = ____ oz = ____ cup

67. 99.5°F = ____ °C

Chapter 2 Post-Test: Systems of Measurement and Common Equivalents

Name _____ **Date** _____

1. 2.2 lb   = ____ kg

2. 16 fl oz   = ____ pt

3. 1 tsp   = ____ mL

4. 15 gr   = ____ g

5. 1 oz   = ____ mL

6. 1000 mcg   = ____ mg

7. 60 mg   = ____ gr

8. 1 pt   = ____ mL

9. ½ tsp   = ____ mL

10. 1000 mg   = ____ g

11. 1 L   = ____ mL

12. 4 qt   = ____ gal

13. 1 tbsp   = ____ tsp

14. 1 cup   = ____ oz

15. 8 oz   = ____ mL

16. 3 tsp   = ____ mL

17. 15 gtt   = ____ M

18. 1 dr   = ____ mL

19. 15 M   = ____ mL

20. 1000 g   = ____ kg

21. Coffee Cup = 240 mL (drank all)
    Juice Glass = 120 mL (drank ½)
    Hot Cereal = 100 mL (ate all)
    Total   =

22. Milk Carton = 120 mL (drank all)
    Soup Bowl   = 100 mL (ate all)
    Jello Cup   = 120 mL (ate ½)
    Total   =

23. 100.4°F   = _____ °C

24. 39.5°C   = _____ °F

25. 96.8°F   = _____°C

26. 35°C   = _____°F

27. 1400 MT   = _____ ST

28. 10:15 pm ST = _____ MT

29. 6:00 am ST   = _____ MT

30. 1630 MT   = _____ ST

ANSWER KEY FOR CHAPTER 2: SYSTEMS OF MEASUREMENT AND COMMON EQUIVALENTS

Practice Problems

1. kilogram   = kg
2. gram   = g
3. milligram   = mg
4. microgram   = mcg
5. liter   = L
6. milliliter   = mL
7. pound   = lb
8. ounce   = oz
9. dram   = dr
10. grain   = gr
11. gallon   = gal
12. quart   = qt
13. pint   = pt
14. fluid ounce   = fl oz
15. fluid dram   = fl dr
16. minim   = M
17. tablespoon   = tbsp
18. teaspoon   = tsp
19. drop   = gtt
20. 1 kg   = 2.2 lb
21. 1 kg   = 1000 g
22. 1 g   = 1000 mg
23. 1 mg   = 1000 mcg
24. 1 g   = 15 gr
25. Breakfast:

Coffee Cup	= 240 mL (drank ½)	120
Water Glass	= 180 mL (drank ½ with AM medications)	90
Juice Glass	= 120 mL (drank all)	120
Hot Cereal	= 100 mL (ate ½)	50
Total	=	380 mL

26. Lunch:

Coffee Cup	= 240 mL (drank all)	240
Small Milk Carton	= 120 mL (drank all)	120
Large Soup Bowl	= 200 mL (ate ½)	100
Jello Cup	= 120 mL (ate all)	120
Total	=	580 mL

27. Dinner:

Coffee Cup	= 240 mL (drank ¼)	60
Large Milk Carton	= 240 mL (drank ½)	120
Ice Cream	= 90 mL (ate all)	90
Total	=	270 mL

28. 98.6°F   = 37°C
29. 39°C   = 102.2°F
30. 104.9°F   = 40.5°C
31. 36°C   = 96.8°F
32. 101.3°F   = 38.5°C

Convert the following Standard Times to Military Time:

33. 1:00 am = 0100
34. 5:00 pm = 1700
35. 3:00 am = 0300
36. 8:00 pm = 2000
37. 12:00 am = 2400

Convert the following Military Times to Standard Time:

38. 0230   = 2:30 am
39. 1600   = 4:00 pm
40. 0420   = 4:20 am
41. 1200   = 12:00 pm
42. 2110   = 9:10 pm
43. 1 gr   = 60 mg
44. 1000 mg = 1 g
45. 1000 mL = 1 L = 1 qt
46. 500 mL   = 1 pt
47. 240 mL   = 8 oz
48. 30 mL   = 1 oz = 2 tbsp
49. 15 mL   = ½ oz = 3 tsp
50. 5 mL   = 1 tsp
51. 1 mL   = 15 M = 15 gtt
52. 2 mL   = 30 gtt
53. 30 gtt   = 30 M = 2 mL
54. 4 tbsp   = 2 oz = 60 mL
55. 40°C   = 104°F
56. 1 pt   = 16 fl oz = 500 mL
57. 2 qt   = ½ gal = 2000 mL
58. 96.8°F   = 36°C
59. 2000 g   = 2 kg = 4.4 lb
60. gr xv   = 1 g = 1000 mg
61. 37.5°C   = 99.5°F
62. 1 oz   = 8 dr = 30 mL
63. 32 fl oz   = 2 pt = 1000 mL
64. 39°C   = 102.2°F
65. gr xxx   = 2 g = 1800 mg
66. 240 mL   = 8 oz = 1 cup
67. 99.5°F   = 37.5°C

CHAPTER **3**

Solving Problems Using Dimensional Analysis

Dimensional analysis provides a systematic, straightforward way to set up problems and to organize and evaluate data. It is not only easy to learn, but also can reduce **medication errors** when mathematical conversion is required.

PREVENTING MEDICATION ERRORS

Dimensional analysis assists with preventing medication errors by allowing you to visualize all parts of the medication problem and to critically think your way through the problem.

This chapter introduces you to dimensional analysis with a step-by-step explanation of this problem-solving method. The chapter also provides the opportunity to practice solving problems that involve common equivalents.

■ TERMS USED IN DIMENSIONAL ANALYSIS

Dimensional analysis is a problem-solving method that can be used whenever two quantities are directly proportional to each other and one quantity must be converted to the other by using a common equivalent, conversion factor, or conversion relation. All medication dosage calculation problems can be solved by dimensional analysis.

It is important to understand the following four terms that provide the basis for dimensional analysis.

- **Given quantity:** the beginning point of the problem
- **Wanted quantity:** the answer to the problem
- **Unit path:** the series of conversions necessary to achieve the answer to the problem
- **Conversion factors:** equivalents necessary to convert between systems of measurement and to allow unwanted units to be canceled from the problem
  Each conversion factor is a ratio of units that equals 1.

Dimensional analysis also uses the same terms as fractions: numerators and denominators.

- *Numerator* = the top portion of the problem
- *Denominator* = the bottom portion of the problem

Some problems will have a given quantity and a wanted quantity that contain only numerators. Other problems will have a given quantity and a wanted quantity that contain both a numerator and a denominator. This chapter contains only problems with numerators as the given quantity and the wanted quantity.

Once the beginning point in the problem is identified, then a series of conversions necessary to achieve the answer is established that leads to the problem's solution.

Below is an example of the model that is used in solving problems by the dimensional analysis method. It also demonstrates the correct placement of the basic terms that are used in this method.

Unit Path

Given Quantity	Conversion Factor for Given Quantity	Conversion Factor for Wanted Quantity	Conversion Computation	Wanted Quantity

■ THE FIVE STEPS OF DIMENSIONAL ANALYSIS

Once the given quantity is identified, the unit path leading to the wanted quantity is established. The problem-solving method of dimensional analysis uses the following five steps.

1. Identify the *given quantity* in the problem.
2. Identify the *wanted quantity* in the problem.

3. Establish the *unit path* from the given quantity to the wanted quantity using equivalents as *conversion factors*.
4. Set up the conversion factors to permit cancellation of unwanted units. Carefully choose each conversion factor and ensure that it is correctly placed in the numerator or denominator portion of the problem to allow the unwanted units to be canceled from the problem.
5. Multiply the numerators, multiply the denominators, and divide the product of the numerators by the product of the denominators to provide the numerical value of the wanted quantity.

The following examples use the five steps to solve problems using dimensional analysis. New information that is added in each step appears in red. Lines show that unwanted units or numbers have been canceled from the unit path. A circle appears around the wanted quantity in the unit path.

EXAMPLE 3.1

▶ **1 liter (L) equals how many ounces (oz)?**

STEP 1 Identify the *given quantity* in the problem.

Unit Path

Given Quantity	Conversion Factor for Given Quantity	Conversion Factor for Wanted Quantity	Conversion Computation	Wanted Quantity
1 liter (L)				=

▶▶▶ *The given quantity is* 1 L.

STEP 2 Identify the *wanted quantity* in the problem.

Unit Path

Given Quantity	Conversion Factor for Given Quantity	Conversion Factor for Wanted Quantity	Conversion Computation	Wanted Quantity
1 liter (L)				= oz

▶▶▶ *The wanted quantity is the number of* ounces (oz) in 1 L.

STEP 3 Establish the *unit path* from the given quantity to the wanted quantity. You must determine what conversion factors are needed to convert the given quantity to the wanted quantity.

▶▶▶ *Given quantity: 1 L = 1000 mL*
Wanted quantity: 1 oz = 30 mL

STEP 4 Write the unit path for the problem so that each unit cancels out the preceding unit until all unwanted units are canceled from the problem except the wanted quantity. Red lines indicate that unwanted units or numbers have been canceled.

    The wanted quantity must be within the numerator portion of the problem. A red circle around the wanted quantity demonstrates that the problem is set up correctly.

Unit Path

Given Quantity	Conversion Factor for Given Quantity	Conversion Factor for Wanted Quantity	Conversion Computation	Wanted Quantity
1 liter (L)	1000 mL	1 oz		
	1 liter (L)	30 mL		= oz

Unit Path

Given Quantity	Conversion Factor for Given Quantity	Conversion Factor for Wanted Quantity	Conversion Computation	Wanted Quantity
1 liter (L)	1000 mL	1 (oz)		
	1 liter (L)	30 mL		= oz

STEP 5 After the unwanted units are canceled from the problem, only the numerical values remain. Multiply the numerators, multiply the denominators, and divide the product of the numerators by the product of the denominators to provide the numerical value for the wanted quantity.

    One (1) times (×) any number equals that number, therefore 1s may be automatically canceled from the problem. Other factors that can be canceled from the problem include like numerical values in the numerator and denominator portion of the problem and the same number of zeroes in the numerator and denominator portion of the problem.

Unit Path

Given Quantity	Conversion Factor for Given Quantity	Conversion Factor for Wanted Quantity	Conversion Computation		Wanted Quantity
1 liter (L)	1000 mL	1 (oz)	1000 × 1	1000	
	1 liter (L)	30 mL	1 × 30	30	= 33.3 oz

▶ ▶ ▶ *33.3 oz is the wanted quantity and the answer to the problem.*

EXAMPLE 3.2

▶ **One gallon (gal) equals how many milliliters (mL)?**

STEP 1 Identify the given quantity in the problem.

$$\frac{1 \text{ gal} \quad}{\quad} =$$

▶▶▶ *The given quantity is 1 gal.*

STEP 2 Identify the wanted quantity in the problem.

$$\frac{1 \text{ gal} \quad}{\quad} = \text{mL}$$

▶▶▶ *The wanted quantity is the number of milliliters (mL) in 1 gal.*

STEP 3 Establish the unit path from the given quantity to the wanted quantity by selecting the equivalents that will be used as conversion factors.

▶▶▶ *Given quantity: 1 gal = 4 quarts (qt); 1 qt = 1 L*
Wanted quantity: 1 L = 1000 mL

STEP 4 Write the unit path for the problem so that each unit cancels out (red lines) the preceding unit until all unwanted units are canceled from the problem except the wanted quantity, which is circled.

$$\frac{1 \text{ gal} \;\left|\; 4 \text{ qt} \;\left|\; 1 \text{ L} \;\left|\; 1000 \text{ (mL)}\right.\right.\right.}{\left.\left|\; 1 \text{ gal} \;\left|\; 1 \text{ qt} \;\left|\; 1 \text{ L}\right.\right.\right.} = \quad \text{mL}$$

STEP 5 After the unwanted units are canceled from the problem, only the numerical values remain. Multiply the numerators, multiply the denominators, and divide the product of the numerators by the product of the denominators to provide the numerical value for the wanted quantity.

$$\frac{1 \text{ gal} \;\left|\; 4 \text{ qt} \;\left|\; 1 \text{ L} \;\left|\; 1000 \text{ (mL)} \;\left|\; 4 \times 1000\right.\right.\right.\right.}{\left.\left|\; 1 \text{ gal} \;\left|\; 1 \text{ qt} \;\left|\; 1 \text{ L} \;\left|\; 1\right.\right.\right.\right.} = 4000 \text{ mL}$$

▶▶▶ *4000 mL is the wanted quantity and the answer to the problem.*

Exercise 3.1	**Dimensional Analysis**
	(See pages 59–61 for answers)

Use dimensional analysis to change the following units of measurement.

1. Problem: 4 mg = How many g?

   Given quantity   =

   Wanted quantity   =

   $$\frac{4 \text{ mg}}{\qquad\qquad\qquad\qquad\qquad\qquad} = \qquad \text{g}$$

2. Problem: 5000 g = How many kg?

   Given quantity   =

   Wanted quantity   =

   $$\frac{5000 \text{ g}}{\qquad\qquad\qquad\qquad\qquad\qquad} = \qquad \text{kg}$$

3. Problem: 0.3 L = How many mL?

   Given quantity   =

   Wanted quantity   =

   $$\frac{0.3 \text{ L}}{\qquad\qquad\qquad\qquad\qquad\qquad} = \qquad \text{mL}$$

4. Problem: 15 mL = How many tsp?

   Given quantity   =

   Wanted quantity   =

   $$\frac{15 \text{ mL}}{\qquad\qquad\qquad\qquad\qquad\qquad} = \qquad \text{tsp}$$

5. Problem: 120 lb = How many kg?

   Given quantity   =

   Wanted quantity   =

   $$\frac{120 \text{ lb}}{\qquad\qquad\qquad\qquad\qquad\qquad} = \qquad \text{kg}$$

(Exercise continues on page 52)

6. Problem: 5 gr = How many mg?

   Given quantity   =

   Wanted quantity   =

   $$\frac{5\ gr}{} \underline{\hspace{8cm}} = \quad mg$$

7. Problem: 2 g = How many gr?

   Given quantity   =

   Wanted quantity   =

   $$\frac{2\ g}{} \underline{\hspace{8cm}} = \quad gr$$

8. Problem: 5 fl dr = How many mL?

   Given quantity   =

   Wanted quantity   =

   $$\frac{5\ fl\ dr}{} \underline{\hspace{8cm}} = \quad mL$$

9. Problem: 8 fl dr = How many fl oz?

   Given quantity   =

   Wanted quantity   =

   $$\frac{8\ fl\ dr}{} \underline{\hspace{8cm}} = \quad fl\ oz$$

10. Problem: 10 M = How many fl dr?

    Given quantity   =

    Wanted quantity   =

    $$\frac{10\ M}{} \underline{\hspace{8cm}} = \quad fl\ dr$$

11. Problem: 35 kg = How many lb?

    Given quantity   =

    Wanted quantity   =

    $$\frac{35\ kg}{} \underline{\hspace{8cm}} = \quad lb$$

12. Problem: 10 mL = How many tsp?

   Given quantity   =

   Wanted quantity   =

$$\frac{10\ mL\ \big|}{\big|} \rule{5cm}{0.4pt} = \quad tsp$$

13. Problem: 30 mL = How many tbsp?

   Given quantity   =

   Wanted quantity   =

$$\frac{30\ mL\ \big|}{\big|} \rule{5cm}{0.4pt} = \quad tbsp$$

14. Problem: 0.25 g = How many mg?

   Given quantity   =

   Wanted quantity   =

$$\frac{0.25\ g\ \big|}{\big|} \rule{5cm}{0.4pt} = \quad mg$$

15. Problem: 350 mcg = How many mg?

   Given quantity   =

   Wanted quantity   =

$$\frac{350\ mcg\ \big|}{\big|} \rule{5cm}{0.4pt} = \quad mg$$

16. Problem: 0.75 L = How many mL?

   Given quantity   =

   Wanted quantity   =

$$\frac{0.75\ L\ \big|}{\big|} \rule{5cm}{0.4pt} = \quad mL$$

(Exercise continues on page 54)

17. Problem: 3 hr = How many minutes?

    Given quantity   =

    Wanted quantity   =

    $$\frac{3 \text{ hr}}{} = \quad \text{min}$$

18. Problem: 3.5 mL = How many M?

    Given quantity   =

    Wanted quantity   =

    $$\frac{3.5 \text{ mL}}{} = \quad \text{M}$$

19. Problem: 500 mcg = How many mg?

    Given quantity   =

    Wanted quantity   =

    $$\frac{500 \text{ mcg}}{} = \quad \text{mg}$$

20. Problem: 225 M = How many tsp?

    Given quantity   =

    Wanted quantity   =

    $$\frac{225 \text{ M}}{} = \quad \text{tsp}$$

21. Problem: 2 gal = How many mL?

    Given quantity   =

    Wanted quantity   =

    $$\frac{2 \text{ gal}}{} = \quad \text{mL}$$

22. Problem: 8 pt = How many gal?

    Given quantity   =

    Wanted quantity   =

    $$\frac{8 \text{ pt}}{} = \quad \text{gal}$$

23. Problem: 16 oz = How many mL?

    Given quantity   =

    Wanted quantity   =

    $$\frac{16\ oz}{\rule{1.5cm}{0.4pt}}\rule{8cm}{0.4pt} = \qquad mL$$

24. Problem: 2 cup = How many mL?

    Given quantity   =

    Wanted quantity   =

    $$\frac{2\ cup}{\rule{1.5cm}{0.4pt}}\rule{8cm}{0.4pt} = \qquad mL$$

25. Problem: 2.5 kg = How many g?

    Given quantity   =

    Wanted quantity   =

    $$\frac{2.5\ kg}{\rule{1.5cm}{0.4pt}}\rule{8cm}{0.4pt} = \qquad g$$

Summary

This chapter has introduced you to dimensional analysis with a step-by-step explanation and an opportunity to practice solving problems involving common equivalents. To demonstrate your understanding of dimensional analysis and conversions between systems of measurement, complete the following practice problems.

Practice Problems for Chapter 3	Solving Problems Using Dimensional Analysis (See pages 61–63 for answers)

1. Problem: $\frac{3}{4}$ mL   = How many M?

2. Problem: gtt XV   = How many M?

3. Problem: $\frac{5}{6}$ gr   = How many mg?

4. Problem: How many mL in 3 oz?

5. Problem: 0.5 mg   = How many mcg?

6. Problem: 35 gtt   = How many mL?

7. Problem: How many mL in 3 qt?

8. Problem: 4 gal   = How many qt?

9. Problem: 1.5 cup   = How many mL?

10. Problem: 24 oz   = How many cups?

11. Problem: 132 lb   = How many kg?

12. Problem: 70 kg   = How many lb?

13. Problem: 750 mcg   = How many mg?

14. Problem: 0.5 L   = How many mL?

15. Problem: 1800 g   = How many kg?

16. Problem: 6000 mL   = How many qt?

17. Problem: 180 mL   = How many oz?

18. Problem: 6 dr   = How many mL?

19. Problem: 0.125 mg   = How many mcg?

20. Problem: 90 M   = How many mL?

21. Problem: 145 lb   = How many kg?

22. Problem: $\frac{3}{4}$ gr   = How many mg?

23. Problem: 1500 mg   = How many g?

24. Problem: 3 lb   = How many g?

25. Problem: 0.80 mg   = How many mcg?

Chapter 3 Post-Test: Solving Problems Using Dimensional Analysis

Name _____ **Date** _____

Use dimensional analysis to solve the following conversion problems:

1. 2045 g = How many lb?

2. 1/150 gr = How many mg?

3. 0.004 g = How many mcg?

4. 6 tsp = How many dr?

5. 0.5 L = How many pt?

6. How many L in 250 oz?

7. How many tbsp in 30 mL?

8. How many minims in 60 mL?

9. How many g in 45 gr?

10. How many oz in 1800 g?

11. 300 mg = How many gr?

12. How many mg in gr ¼?

13. 20 mL = How many M?

14. How many mcg in 0.75 mg?

15. 1.5 pt = How many mL?

16. How many lb in 84 kg?

17. 1/300 gr = How many mg?

18. How many kg in 165 lb?

19. How many gr in 30 mg?

20. 6500 mcg = How many mg?

21. 24 fl oz = How many mL?

22. 1.89 L = How many mL?

23. How many gal in 64 fl oz?

24. 15 mg = How many mcg?

25. 0.5 L = How many fl oz?

ANSWER KEY FOR CHAPTER 3: SOLVING PROBLEMS USING DIMENSIONAL ANALYSIS

Exercise 3.1 **Dimensional Analysis**

1. Problem: 4 mg = How many g?
   Given quantity   = 4 mg
   Wanted quantity   = g
   Conversion factor = 1 g = 1000 mg

$$\frac{4 \text{ mg}}{} \left| \frac{1 \text{ g}}{1000 \text{ mg}} \right| \frac{4 \times 1}{1000} \left| \frac{4}{1000} \right. = 0.004 \text{ g}$$

2. Problem: 5000 g = How many kg?
   Given quantity   = 5000 g
   Wanted quantity   = kg
   Conversion factor = 1 kg = 1000 g

$$\frac{5000 \text{ g}}{} \left| \frac{1 \text{ kg}}{1000 \text{ g}} \right| \frac{5 \times 1}{1} \left| \frac{5}{1} \right. = 5 \text{ kg}$$

3. Problem: 0.3 L = How many mL?
   Given quantity   = 0.3 L
   Wanted quantity   = mL
   Conversion factor = 1 L = 1000 mL

$$\frac{0.3 \text{ L}}{} \left| \frac{1000 \text{ mL}}{1 \text{ L}} \right| \frac{0.3 \times 1000}{1} \left| \frac{300}{1} \right. = 300 \text{ mL}$$

4. Problem: 15 mL = How many tsp?
   Given quantity   = 15 mL
   Wanted quantity   = tsp
   Conversion factor = 1 tsp = 5 mL

$$\frac{15 \text{ mL}}{} \left| \frac{1 \text{ tsp}}{5 \text{ mL}} \right| \frac{15 \times 1}{5} \left| \frac{15}{5} \right. = 3 \text{ tsp}$$

5. Problem: 120 lb = How many kg?
   Given quantity   = 120 lb
   Wanted quantity   = kg
   Conversion factor = 2.2 lb = 1 kg

$$\frac{120 \text{ lb}}{} \left| \frac{1 \text{ kg}}{2.2 \text{ lb}} \right| \frac{120 \times 1}{2.2} \left| \frac{120}{2.2} \right. = 54.5 \text{ kg}$$

6. Problem: 5 gr = How many mg?
   Given quantity   = 5 gr
   Wanted quantity   = mg
   Conversion factor = 1 gr = 60 mg

$$\frac{5 \text{ gr}}{} \left| \frac{60 \text{ mg}}{1 \text{ gr}} \right| \frac{5 \times 60}{1} \left| \frac{300}{1} \right. = 300 \text{ mg}$$

7. Problem: 2 g = How many gr?
   Given quantity   = 2 g
   Wanted quantity   = gr
   Conversion factor = 1 g = 15 gr

$$\frac{2 \text{ g}}{} \left| \frac{15 \text{ gr}}{1 \text{ g}} \right| \frac{2 \times 15}{1} \left| \frac{30}{1} \right. = 30 \text{ gr}$$

8. Problem: 5 fl dr = How many mL?
   Given quantity   = 5 fl dr
   Wanted quantity   = mL
   Conversion factor = 1 fl dr = 5 mL

$$\frac{5 \text{ fl dr}}{} \left| \frac{5 \text{ mL}}{1 \text{ fl dr}} \right| \frac{5 \times 5}{1} \left| \frac{25}{1} \right. = 25 \text{ mL}$$

9. Problem: 8 fl dr = How many fl oz?
   Given quantity   = 8 fl dr
   Wanted quantity   = fl oz
   Conversion factor = 1 fl dr = 5 mL
   Conversion factor = 1 fl oz = 30 mL

$$\frac{8 \text{ fl dr}}{} \left| \frac{5 \text{ mL}}{1 \text{ fl dr}} \right| \frac{1 \text{ fl oz}}{30 \text{ mL}} \left| \frac{8 \times 5 \times 1}{1 \times 30} \right| \frac{40}{30} = 1.3 \text{ fl oz}$$

10. Problem: 10 M = How many fl dr?
    Given quantity   = M
    Wanted quantity   = fl dr
    Conversion factor = 1 mL = 15 M
    Conversion factor = 1 fl dr = 5 mL

$$\frac{10 \text{ M}}{} \left| \frac{1 \text{ mL}}{15 \text{ M}} \right| \frac{1 \text{ fl dr}}{5 \text{ mL}} \left| \frac{10 \times 1 \times 1}{15 \times 5} \right| \frac{10}{75} = 0.13 \text{ fl dr}$$

11. Problem: 35 kg = How many lb?
    Given quantity   = 35 kg
    Wanted quantity   = lb
    Conversion factor = 1 kg = 2.2 lb

$$\frac{35\ kg}{} \left| \frac{2.2\ \text{(lb)}}{1\ kg} \right| \frac{35 \times 2.2}{1} \left| \frac{77}{1} \right. = 77\ lb$$

12. Problem: 10 mL = How many tsp?
    Given quantity   = 10 mL
    Wanted quantity   = tsp
    Conversion factor = 1 tsp = 5 mL

$$\frac{10\ mL}{} \left| \frac{1\ \text{(tsp)}}{5\ mL} \right| \frac{10 \times 1}{5} \left| \frac{10}{5} \right. = 2\ tsp$$

13. Problem: 30 mL = How many tbsp?
    Given quantity   = 30 mL
    Wanted quantity   = tbsp
    Conversion factor = 1 tbsp = 15 mL

$$\frac{30\ mL}{} \left| \frac{1\ \text{(tbsp)}}{15\ mL} \right| \frac{30 \times 1}{15} \left| \frac{30}{15} \right. = 2\ tbsp$$

14. Problem: 0.25 g = How many mg?
    Given quantity   = 0.25 g
    Wanted quantity   = mg
    Conversion factor = 1 g = 1000 mg

$$\frac{0.25\ g}{} \left| \frac{1000\ \text{(mg)}}{1\ g} \right| \frac{0.25 \times 1000}{1} \left| \frac{250}{1} \right. = 250\ mg$$

15. Problem: 350 mcg = How many mg?
    Given quantity   = 350 mcg
    Wanted quantity   = mg
    Conversion factor = 1 mg = 1000 mcg

$$\frac{350\ mcg}{} \left| \frac{1\ \text{(mg)}}{1000\ mcg} \right| \frac{350 \times 1}{1000} \left| \frac{350}{1000} \right. = 0.35\ mg$$

16. Problem: 0.75 L = How many mL?
    Given quantity   = 0.75 L
    Wanted quantity   = mL
    Conversion factor = 1 L = 1000 mL

$$\frac{0.75\ L}{} \left| \frac{1000\ \text{(mL)}}{1\ L} \right| \frac{0.75 \times 1000}{1} \left| \frac{750}{1} \right. = 750\ mL$$

17. Problem: 3 hr = How many minutes?
    Given quantity   = 3 hr
    Wanted quantity   = minutes
    Conversion factor = 1 hr = 60 min

$$\frac{3\ hr}{} \left| \frac{60\ \text{(min)}}{1\ hr} \right| \frac{3 \times 60}{1} \left| \frac{180}{1} \right. = 180\ min$$

18. Problem: 3.5 mL = How many M?
    Given quantity   = 3.5 mL
    Wanted quantity   = M
    Conversion factor = 1 mL = 15 M

$$\frac{3.5\ mL}{} \left| \frac{15\ \text{(M)}}{1\ mL} \right| \frac{3.5 \times 15}{1} \left| \frac{52.5}{1} \right. = 52.5\ M$$

19. Problem: 500 mcg = How many mg?
    Given quantity   = 500 mcg
    Wanted quantity   = mg
    Conversion factor = 1 mg = 1000 mcg

$$\frac{500\ mcg}{} \left| \frac{1\ \text{(mg)}}{1000\ mcg} \right| \frac{500 \times 1}{1000} \left| \frac{500}{1000} \right. = 0.5\ mg$$

20. Problem: 225 M = How many tsp?
    Given quantity   = 225 M
    Wanted quantity   = tsp
    Conversion factor = 1 mL = 15 M
    Conversion factor = 1 tsp = 5 mL

$$\frac{225\ M}{} \left| \frac{1\ mL}{15\ M} \right| \frac{1\ \text{(tsp)}}{5\ mL} \left| \frac{225 \times 1 \times 1}{15 \times 5} \right| \frac{225}{75} = 3\ tsp$$

21. Problem: 2 gal = How many mL?
    Given quantity = gal
    Wanted quantity = mL
    Conversion factor = 1 gal = 4000 mL

$$\frac{2 \text{ gal} \mid 4000 \text{ (mL)} \mid 2 \times 4000 \mid 8000}{1 \text{ gal} \mid 1 \mid 1} = 8000 \text{ mL}$$

22. Problem: 8 pt = How man gal?
    Given quantity = pt
    Wanted quantity = gal
    Conversion factor = 1 qt = 2 pt
    Conversion factor = 1 gal = 4 qt

$$\frac{8 \text{ pt} \mid 1 \text{ qt} \mid 1 \text{ (gal)} \mid 8 \times 1 \times 1 \mid 8}{2 \text{ pt} \mid 4 \text{ qt} \mid 2 \times 4 \mid 8} = 1 \text{ gal}$$

23. Problem: 16 oz = How many mL?
    Given quantity = oz
    Wanted quantity = mL
    Conversion factor = 1 oz = 30 mL

$$\frac{16 \text{ oz} \mid 30 \text{ (mL)} \mid 16 \times 30 \mid 480}{1 \text{ oz} \mid 1 \mid 1} = 480 \text{ mL}$$

24. Problem: 2 cup = How many mL?
    Given quantity = cup
    Wanted quantity = mL
    Conversion factor = 1 cup = 8 oz
    Conversion factor = 8 oz = 240 mL

$$\frac{2 \text{ cup} \mid 8 \text{ oz} \mid 240 \text{ (mL)} \mid 2 \times 8 \times 240 \mid 3840}{1 \text{ cup} \mid 8 \text{ oz} \mid 1 \times 8 \mid 8} = 480 \text{ mL}$$

25. Problem: 2.5 kg = How many g?
    Given quantity = kg
    Wanted quantity = g
    Conversion factor = 1 kg = 1000 g

$$\frac{2.5 \text{ kg} \mid 1000 \text{ (g)} \mid 2.5 \times 1000 \mid 2500}{1 \text{ kg} \mid 1 \mid 1} = 2500 \text{ g}$$

Practice Problems

1. Problem: $\frac{3}{4}$ mL = How many M?
   Given quantity = $\frac{3}{4}$ mL
   Wanted quantity = M
   Conversion factor = 1 mL = 15 M

$$\frac{\frac{3}{4} \text{ mL} \mid 15 \text{ (M)} \mid \frac{3}{4} \times 15 \mid \frac{3}{4} \times \frac{15}{1} \mid \frac{45}{4} \mid 11.25 \text{ M}}{1 \text{ mL} \mid 1 \mid 1 \mid 1 \mid 1} = 11.25 \text{ M}$$

2. Problem: gtt XV = How many M?
   Given quantity = 15 gtt
   Wanted quantity = M
   Conversion factor = 1 gtt = 1 M

$$\frac{15 \text{ gtt} \mid 1 \text{ (M)} \mid 15}{1 \text{ gtt} \mid} = 15 \text{ M}$$

3. Problem: $\frac{5}{6}$ gr = How many mg?
   Given quantity = $\frac{5}{6}$ gr
   Wanted quantity = mg
   Conversion factor = 1 gr = 60 mg

$$\frac{\frac{5}{6} \text{ gr} \mid 60 \text{ (mg)} \mid \frac{5}{6} \times 60 \mid \frac{5}{6} \times \frac{60}{1} \mid \frac{300}{6} \mid 50}{1 \text{ gr} \mid 1 \mid 1 \mid 1 \mid 1} = 50 \text{ mg}$$

4. Problem: How many mL in 3 oz?
   Given quantity = 3 oz
   Wanted quantity = mL
   Conversion factor = 1 oz = 30 mL

$$\frac{3 \text{ oz} \mid 30 \text{ (mL)} \mid 3 \times 30 \mid 90}{1 \text{ oz} \mid 1 \mid 1} = 90 \text{ mL}$$

5. Problem: 0.5 mg = How many mcg?
   Given quantity = 0.5 mg
   Wanted quantity = mcg
   Conversion factor = 1 mg = 1000 mcg

$$\frac{0.5 \text{ mg} \mid 1000 \text{ (mcg)} \mid 0.5 \times 1000 \mid 500}{1 \text{ mg} \mid 1 \mid 1} = 500 \text{ mcg}$$

6. Problem: 35 gtt = How many mL?
   Given quantity   = 35 gtt
   Wanted quantity   = mL
   Conversion factor = 1 gtt = 1 M
   Conversion factor = 15 M = 1 mL

$$\frac{35 \text{ gtt}}{} \left| \frac{1\text{M}}{1 \text{ gtt}} \right| \frac{1 \text{ mL}}{15 \text{ M}} \left| \frac{35 \times 1 \times 1}{1 \times 15} \right| \frac{35}{15} = 2.3 \text{ mL}$$

7. Problem: How many mL in 3 qt?
   Given quantity   = 3 qt
   Wanted quantity   = mL
   Conversion factor = 1 qt = 1000 mL
   Conversion factor = 1 cc = 1 mL

$$\frac{3 \text{ qt}}{} \left| \frac{1000 \text{ mL}}{1 \text{ qt}} \right| \frac{3 \times 1000}{1} \left| \frac{3000}{1} \right. = 3000 \text{ mL}$$

8. Problem: 4 gal = How many qt?
   Given quantity   = 4 gal
   Wanted quantity   = qt
   Conversion factor = 1 gal = 4 qt

$$\frac{4 \text{ gal}}{} \left| \frac{4 \text{ qt}}{1 \text{ gal}} \right| \frac{4 \times 4}{1} \left| \frac{16}{1} \right. = 16 \text{ qt}$$

9. Problem: 1.5 cup = How many mL?
   Given quantity   = 1.5 cup
   Wanted quantity   = mL
   Conversion factor = 1 cup = 240 mL

$$\frac{1.5 \text{ cup}}{} \left| \frac{240 \text{ mL}}{1 \text{ cup}} \right| \frac{1.5 \times 240}{1} \left| \frac{360}{1} \right. = 360 \text{ mL}$$

10. Problem: 24 oz = How many cups?
    Given quantity   = 24 oz
    Wanted quantity   = cups
    Conversion factor = 1 cup = 8 oz

$$\frac{24 \text{ oz}}{} \left| \frac{1 \text{ cup}}{8 \text{ oz}} \right| \frac{24 \times 1}{8} \left| \frac{24}{8} \right. = 3 \text{ cups}$$

11. Problem: 132 lb = How many kg?
    Given quantity   = 132 lb
    Wanted quantity   = kg
    Conversion factor = 2.2 lb = 1 kg

$$\frac{132 \text{ lb}}{} \left| \frac{1 \text{ kg}}{2.2 \text{ lb}} \right| \frac{132 \times 1}{2.2} \left| \frac{132}{2.2} \right. = 60 \text{ kg}$$

12. Problem: 70 kg = How many lb?
    Given quantity   = 70 kg
    Wanted quantity   = lb
    Conversion factor = 1 kg = 2.2 lb

$$\frac{70 \text{ kg}}{} \left| \frac{2.2 \text{ lb}}{1 \text{ kg}} \right| \frac{70 \times 2.2}{1} \left| \frac{154}{1} \right. = 154 \text{ lb}$$

13. Problem: 750 mcg = How many mg?
    Given quantity   = 750 mcg
    Wanted quantity   = mg
    Conversion factor = 1000 mcg = 1 mL

$$\frac{750 \text{ mcg}}{} \left| \frac{1 \text{ mg}}{1000 \text{ mcg}} \right| \frac{75 \times 1}{100} \left| \frac{75}{100} \right. = 0.75 \text{ mg}$$

14. Problem: 0.5 L = How many mL?
    Given quantity   = 0.5 L
    Wanted quantity   = mL
    Conversion factor = 1 L = 1000 mL

$$\frac{0.5 \text{ L}}{} \left| \frac{1000 \text{ mL}}{1 \text{ L}} \right| \frac{0.5 \times 1000}{1} \left| \frac{500}{1} \right. = 500 \text{ mL}$$

15. Problem: 1800 g = How many kg?
    Given quantity   = 1800 g
    Wanted quantity   = kg
    Conversion factor = 1000 g = 1 kg

$$\frac{1800 \text{ g}}{} \left| \frac{1 \text{ kg}}{1000 \text{ g}} \right| \frac{18 \times 1}{10} \left| \frac{18}{10} \right. = 1.8 \text{ kg}$$

16. Problem: How many qt in 6000 mL?
    Given quantity   = 6000 mL
    Wanted quantity   = qt
    Conversion factor = 1000 mL = 1 qt

$$\frac{6000 \text{ mL} \quad | \quad 1 \text{ qt} \quad | \quad 6000 \times 1 \quad | \quad 6000}{\qquad\qquad | \quad 1000 \text{ mL} \quad | \quad 1000 \quad | \quad 1000} = 6 \text{ qt}$$

17. Problem: 180 mL = How many oz?
    Given quantity   = 180 mL
    Wanted quantity   = oz
    Conversion factor = 30 mL = 1 oz

$$\frac{180 \text{ mL} \quad | \quad 1 \text{ oz} \quad | \quad 18 \times 1 \quad | \quad 18}{\qquad\qquad | \quad 30 \text{ mL} \quad | \quad 3 \quad | \quad 3} = 6 \text{ oz}$$

18. Problem: 6 dr = How many mL?
    Given quantity   = 6 dr
    Wanted quantity   = mL
    Conversion factor = 1 dr = 5 mL

$$\frac{6 \text{ dr} \quad | \quad 5 \text{ mL} \quad | \quad 6 \times 5 \quad | \quad 30}{\qquad | \quad 1 \text{ dr} \quad | \quad 1 \quad | \quad 1} = 30 \text{ mL}$$

19. Problem: 0.125 mg = How many mcg?
    Given quantity   = 0.125 mg
    Wanted quantity   = mcg
    Conversion factor = 1 mg = 1000 mcg

$$\frac{0.125 \text{ mg} \quad | \quad 1000 \text{ mcg} \quad | \quad 0.125 \times 1000 \quad | \quad 125}{\qquad\qquad | \quad 1 \text{ mg} \quad | \quad 1 \quad | \quad 1} = 125 \text{ mcg}$$

20. Problem: How many mL in 90 M?
    Given quantity   = 90 M
    Wanted quantity   = mL
    Conversion factor =

$$\frac{90 \text{ M} \quad | \quad 1 \text{ mL} \quad | \quad 90 \times 1 \quad | \quad 90}{\qquad | \quad 15 \text{ M} \quad | \quad 15 \quad | \quad 15} = 6 \text{ mL}$$

21. Problem: 145 lb = How many kg?
    Given quantity   = 145 lb
    Wanted quantity   = kg
    Conversion factor = 1 kg = 2.2 lb

$$\frac{145 \text{ lb} \quad | \quad 1 \text{ kg} \quad | \quad 145 \times 1 \quad | \quad 145}{\qquad\qquad | \quad 2.2 \text{ lb} \quad | \quad 2.2 \quad | \quad 2.2} = 65.9 \text{ kg}$$

22. Problem: $\frac{3}{4}$ gr = How many mg?
    Given quantity   = $\frac{3}{4}$ gr
    Wanted quantity   = mg
    Conversion factor = 1 gr = 60 mg

$$\frac{\frac{3}{4} \text{ gr} \quad | \quad 60 \text{ mg} \quad | \quad \frac{3}{4} \times \frac{60}{1} \quad | \quad \frac{180}{4} \quad | \quad 45}{\qquad\qquad | \quad 1 \text{ gr} \quad | \quad 1 \quad | \quad 1 \quad | \quad 1} = 45 \text{ mg}$$

23. Problem: How many g in 1500 mg?
    Given quantity   = 1500 mg
    Wanted quantity   = g
    Conversion factor = 1 g = 1000 mg

$$\frac{1500 \text{ mg} \quad | \quad 1 \text{ g} \quad | \quad 1500 \times 1 \quad | \quad 1500}{\qquad\qquad | \quad 1000 \text{ mg} \quad | \quad 1000 \quad | \quad 1000} = 15 \text{ g}$$

24. Problem: 3 lb = How many g?
    Given quantity   = 3 lb
    Wanted quantity   = g
    Conversion factor = 2.2 lb = 1000 g

$$\frac{3 \text{ lb} \quad | \quad 1000 \text{ g} \quad | \quad 3 \times 1000 \quad | \quad 3000}{\qquad | \quad 2.2 \text{ lb} \quad | \quad 2.2 \quad | \quad 2.2} = 1363.6 \text{ g}$$

25. Problem: 0.80 mg = How many mcg?
    Given quantity   = 0.80 mg
    Wanted quantity   = mcg
    Conversion factor = 1 mg = 1000 mcg

$$\frac{0.80 \text{ mg} \quad | \quad 1000 \text{ mcg} \quad | \quad 0.80 \times 1000 \quad | \quad 800}{\qquad\qquad | \quad 1 \text{ mg} \quad | \quad 1 \quad | \quad 1} = 800 \text{ mcg}$$

CHAPTER 4

One-Factor
Medication Problems

Objectives

After completing this chapter, you will successfully be able to:

1. Interpret medication orders correctly, based on the six rights of medication administration.
2. Identify components from a drug label that are needed for accurate medication administration and documentation.
3. Describe the different routes of medication administration: tablets and capsules, liquids given by medicine cup or syringe, and parenteral injections using different types of syringes.
4. Calculate medication problems accurately from the one-factor–given quantity to the one-factor–wanted quantity using the sequential or random method of dimensional analysis.

Outline

For accurate administration of medication, the six rights of medication administration form the foundation of communication between the person writing the medication order and the person reading the medication order.

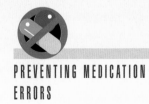

PREVENTING MEDICATION ERRORS

The physician or nurse practitioner writes a medication order using the six rights, and the nurse administers the medication to the patient based on the six rights. There may be a slight variation in the way each person writes a medication order, but information pertaining to the six rights should be included in the medication order to ensure safe administration by the nurse and the prevention of **medication errors.**

To calculate the change from a one-factor-given quantity to a one-factor-wanted quantity using dimensional analysis, it is necessary to have a clear understanding of the six rights of medication administration. This chapter teaches you to interpret medication orders correctly and to calculate medication problems accurately using dimensional analysis.

■ INTERPRETATION OF MEDICATION ORDERS

Physicians and nurse practitioners order medications using the **six rights** of medication administration including the:

1. Right **patient**
2. Right **drug**
3. Right **dosage**

4. Right **route**
5. Right **time**
6. Right **documentation**

Right Patient

Many medication errors can be prevented by correctly identifying the **right patient.** Patients in the hospital setting wear identification bands, whereas other facilities may use a photograph to identify the **right patient.**

Regardless of the identification method, the medication order must correspond to the identification of the patient. Checking identification and asking patients to state their names assists in reducing medication errors. It is also important to "listen" to the patient. If the patient states, "I don't take a blue pill," go back and check the medication order for correctness.

Right Drug

Medications can be ordered using their **trade name** or **generic name.**
Examples:

1. Tagamet® or cimetidine
2. Cipro® or ciprofloxacin hydrochloride

It is the responsibility of the nurse to look up a medication before administration to ensure that the **right drug** is being administered.

It is the responsibility of the nurse to know the classification of the drug being administered and that the drug corresponds with the patient diagnosis. Many drugs have similar names.
Example:

1. Celebrex® (an anti-inflammatory)
2. Celexa® (an antidepressant)

It is also the responsibility of the nurse to know the side effects of the drug being administered. The nurse must be aware of any patient allergies before medication administration to ensure safety of the patient. Allergies should be clearly recorded on medication records or a patient should wear an allergy bracelet.

PREVENTING MEDICATION ERRORS

Medication errors can be prevented by carefully adhering to these **six rights,** understanding the important concepts that apply to each right, and utilizing a nursing drug reference to provide accurate information for each medication administered.

Once you are able to interpret the important components of a medication order, you can perform accurate calculations for the correct dosage using dimensional analysis. If you cannot correctly interpret the components of a medication order (illegible prescription order), call the physician or nurse practitioner for clarification to prevent **medication errors.**

THINKING IT THROUGH

Both *10 gr* and *tablets* are numerators without a denominator. This is called a **one-factor** medication problem because the given quantity and the wanted quantity contain only numerators.

The dose on hand (5 gr/ tablet) is an equivalent that is used as a conversion factor and is factored into the unit path.

The unwanted units (gr) can be canceled from the problem leaving the wanted quantity (tablets) in the numerator.

The **sequential method** of dimensional analysis has been used to factor in the dose on hand, which allows the previous unit (given quantity) to be canceled. When using the sequential method, the conversion factor that is factored in always cancels out the preceding unit.

EXAMPLE 4.1

The physician orders gr 10 aspirin orally every 4 hours, as needed for fever. The unit dose of medication on hand is gr 5 per tablet (5 gr/tab).

▶ **How many tablets will you administer?**

Given quantity   = 10 gr
Wanted quantity = tablets
Dose on hand   = gr/tablet

STEP 1 Identify the *given quantity* (the physician's order).

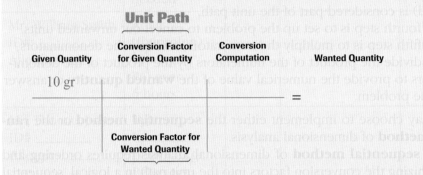

STEP 2 Identify the *wanted quantity* (the answer to the problem).

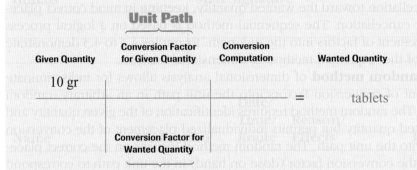

STEP 3 Establish the unit path from the given quantity to the wanted quantity using equivalents as conversion factors.

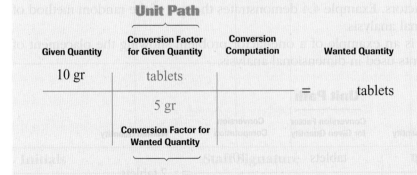

STEP 4 Set up the problem to allow cancellation of unwanted units and circle the wanted quantity within the unit path to demonstrate correct placement.

Unit Path

Given Quantity	Conversion Factor for Given Quantity	Conversion Computation	Wanted Quantity

$$\frac{10\,\text{gr}}{} \cdot \frac{\boxed{\text{tablets}}}{5\,\text{gr}} = \text{tablets}$$

Conversion Factor for Wanted Quantity

STEP 5 Multiply the numerators, multiply the denominators, and divide the product of the numerators by the product of the denominators to provide the numerical value for the wanted quantity.

Unit Path

Given Quantity	Conversion Factor for Given Quantity	Conversion Computation	Wanted Quantity

$$\frac{10\,\text{gr}}{} \cdot \frac{\boxed{\text{tablets}}}{5\,\text{gr}} \cdot \frac{10}{5} = 2\ \text{tablets}$$

Conversion Factor for Wanted Quantity

▶▶▶ *2 tablets is the wanted quantity and the answer to the problem.*

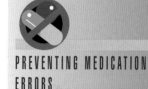

EXAMPLE 4.2

Administer PO Advil (ibuprofen) 400 mg every 6 hours for arthritis. The dosage on hand is 200 mg/tablet.

▶ **How many tablets will you give?**

Given quantity = 400 mg
Wanted quantity = tablets
Dose on hand = 200 mg/tablet

STEP 1 Identify the *given quantity.*

$$\frac{400\ \text{mg}}{} \bigg| =$$

(Example continues on page 72)

STEP 2 Identify the *wanted quantity*.

$$\frac{400 \text{ mg}}{} = \text{tablets}$$

STEP 3 Establish the unit path from the given quantity to the wanted quantity using equivalents as conversion factors.

$$\frac{400 \text{ mg}}{} \left| \frac{\text{tablet}}{200 \text{ mg}} \right. = \text{tablets}$$

STEP 4 Set up the problem to allow cancellation of unwanted units and circle the wanted quantity within the unit path to demonstrate correct placement.

$$\frac{400 \text{ mg}}{} \left| \frac{\boxed{\text{tablet}}}{200 \text{ mg}} \right. = \text{tablets}$$

STEP 5 Multiply the numerators, multiply the denominators, and divide the product of the numerators by the product of the denominators to provide the numerical value of the wanted quantity.

$$\frac{400 \text{ mg}}{} \left| \frac{\boxed{\text{tablet}}}{200 \text{ mg}} \right| \frac{4}{2} = 2 \text{ tablets}$$

▶ ▶ ▶ *2 tablets is the wanted quantity and the answer to the problem.*

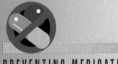

PREVENTING MEDICATION ERRORS

Understanding the principles of rounding will prevent over- or undermedication, both of which are classified as **medication errors.**

Principles of Rounding

If an answer does not result in a whole number, but instead a decimal in the tenths (4.7) or hundredths (4.75), the answer can be rounded up or down to allow for administration of the medication. Some medications may not require rounding when the exact amount of medication calculated needs to be administered.

If the tablets are scored, a half of the tablet can be administered. If a tablet is not scored, a decision must be made by the nurse whether to give one or two tablets. If a liquid medication to be administered involves decimals, then the nurse must make a decision regarding the amount of medication to be given.

If the number following the decimal is 5 or greater, then the number is rounded up.
Example in the tenths: 4.7 → 5
Example in the hundredths: 4.75 → 4.8

If the number following the decimal is less than 5, then the number is rounded down.
Example in the tenths: 4.4 → 4
Example in the hundredths: 4.42 → 4.4

EXAMPLE 4.3

Tylenol (acetaminophen) gr 10 PO every 4 hours for headache. The unit dose of medication on hand is 325 mg per caplet.

▶ **How many caplets will you give?**

Given quantity   = 10 gr
Wanted quantity = caplets
Dose on hand   = 325 mg/caplet

STEP 1 Identify the *given quantity.*

$$\frac{10 \text{ gr}}{\rule{0pt}{2em}} \qquad\qquad\qquad\qquad\qquad =$$

STEP 2 Identify the *wanted quantity.*

$$\frac{10 \text{ gr}}{\rule{0pt}{2em}} \qquad\qquad\qquad\qquad = \text{caplets}$$

STEP 3 Establish the *unit path* from the given quantity to the wanted quantity using equivalents as conversion factors.

$$\frac{10 \text{ gr}}{} \left| \frac{60 \text{ mg}}{1 \text{ gr}} \right| \frac{\text{caplet}}{325 \text{ mg}} = \text{caplets}$$

STEP 4 Set up the problem to allow cancellation of unwanted units and circle the wanted quantity within the unit path to demonstrate correct placement.

$$\frac{10 \text{ gr}}{} \left| \frac{60 \text{ mg}}{1 \text{ gr}} \right| \frac{\boxed{\text{caplet}}}{325 \text{ mg}} = \text{caplets}$$

STEP 5 Multiply the numerators, multiply the denominators, and divide the product of the numerators by the product of the denominators to provide the numerical value of the wanted quantity.

$$\frac{10 \text{ gr}}{} \left| \frac{60 \text{ mg}}{1 \text{ gr}} \right| \frac{\boxed{\text{caplet}}}{325 \text{ mg}} \left| \frac{10 \times 60}{1 \times 325} \right| \frac{600}{325} = 1.8 \text{ caplets}$$

▶▶▶ *1.8 caplets is the wanted quantity and the answer to the problem, but, by using the rounding rule, 2 caplets would be given.*

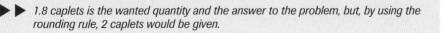

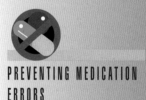

PREVENTING MEDICATION ERRORS

Following the principles of rounding, two caplets would be given as the correct dosage of medication.

Dimensional analysis is a problem-solving method that uses critical thinking, not a specific formula. Therefore, the important concept to remember is that *all* unwanted units must be canceled from the unit path. The **random method** of dimensional analysis can also be used when solving medication problems. When using the random method of dimensional analysis, the focus is on the correct placement of the conversion factor. It must correlate with the wanted quantity in the numerator portion of the unit path, without considering the preceding units.

THINKING IT THROUGH

When using the random method, the focus is on the correct placement of the conversion factor to correspond with the wanted quantity. The problem is set up correctly as long as the dose on hand (caplet) correlates with the wanted quantity (caplet), both in the numerator.

A conversion factor (1 gr = 60 mg) is factored into the problem to cancel out the unwanted units (gr and mg). The remaining unit (caplet) correlates with the wanted quantity.

EXAMPLE 4.4

The random method of dimensional analysis will be used to calculate the answer for Example 4.3.

STEP 1 Identify the *given quantity*.

$$\frac{10 \text{ gr}}{} =$$

STEP 2 Identify the *wanted quantity*.

$$\frac{10 \text{ gr}}{} = \text{caplet}$$

STEP 3 Establish the *unit path* from the given quantity to the wanted quantity using equivalents as conversion factors.

$$\frac{10 \text{ gr}}{} \left| \frac{\text{caplet}}{325 \text{ mg}} \right. = \text{caplet}$$

STEP 4 Set up the problem to allow cancellation of unwanted units and circle the wanted quantity within the unit path to demonstrate correct placement.

$$\frac{10 \text{ \cancel{gr}}}{} \left| \frac{\boxed{\text{caplet}}}{325 \text{ \cancel{mg}}} \right| \frac{60 \text{ \cancel{mg}}}{1 \text{ \cancel{gr}}} = \text{caplet}$$

STEP 5 Multiply the numerators, multiply the denominators, and divide the product of the numerators by the product of the denominators to provide the numerical value of the wanted quantity.

$$\frac{10 \text{ \cancel{gr}}}{} \left| \frac{\boxed{\text{caplet}}}{325 \text{ \cancel{mg}}} \right| \frac{60 \text{ \cancel{mg}}}{1 \text{ \cancel{gr}}} \left| \frac{10 \times 60}{325 \times 1} \right| \frac{600}{325} = 1.8 \text{ caplets}$$

▶▶▶ *1.8 caplets is the wanted quantity and the answer to the problem, but, by using the rounding rule, 2 caplets would be given.*

Exercise 4.3	**One-Factor Medication Problems**

(See pages 105–106 for answers)

1. The physician orders Achromycin (tetracycline) 0.25 g PO every 12 hours for acne. The dosage of medication on hand is 250 mg per capsule.

   ▶ **How many capsules will you give?** _____

2. Administer phenobarbital gr $\frac{1}{2}$ PO tid for sedation. The dosage on hand is 15 mg/tablet.

   ▶ **How many tablets will you give?** _____

3. Give 0.5 g Diuril PO bid for hypertension. Unit dose is 500 mg per tablet.

   ▶ **How many tablets will you give?** _____

4. Order: Restoril 0.03 g PO at bedtime for sedation. Supply: Restoril 30-mg capsules.

   ▶ **How many capsules will you give?** _____

5. Order: Thorazine gr $\frac{1}{2}$ PO tid for singultus. Supply: Thorazine 30-mg capsules.

   ▶ **How many capsules will you give?** _____

■ COMPONENTS OF A DRUG LABEL

All medications (stock and unit dose) are labeled with a drug label that includes specific information to assist in the accurate administration of the medication.

Identifying the Components

Information on the drug label includes:

- Name of the drug, including the trade name (name given by the pharmaceutical company identified with a trademark symbol) and the generic name (chemical name given to the drug)
- Dosage of medication (the amount of medication in each tablet, capsule, or liquid)
- Form of medication (tablet, capsule, or liquid)
- Expiration date (how long the medication will remain stable and safe to administer)
- Lot number or batch number (the manufacturer's batch series for this medication)
- Manufacturer (the pharmaceutical company that produced the medication)

PREVENTING MEDICATION ERRORS

Before administering any medication, the nurse should check the expiration date on the label. Administering a medication that has expired would be considered a **medication error.**

EXAMPLE 4.5

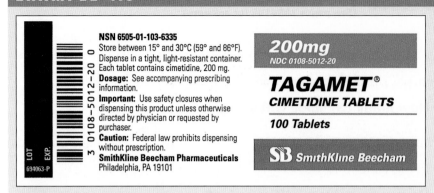

NSN 6505-01-103-6335
Store between 15° and 30°C (59° and 86°F).
Dispense in a tight, light-resistant container.
Each tablet contains cimetidine, 200 mg.
Dosage: See accompanying prescribing
information.
Important: Use safety closures when
dispensing this product unless otherwise
directed by physician or requested by
purchaser.
Caution: Federal law prohibits dispensing
without prescription.
SmithKline Beecham Pharmaceuticals
Philadelphia, PA 19101

200mg
NDC 0108-5012-20

TAGAMET®
CIMETIDINE TABLETS

100 Tablets

SB SmithKline Beecham

Courtesy of SmithKline Beecham Pharmaceuticals.

a. Trade name of the drug: Tagamet
b. Generic name of the drug: Cimetidine
c. Dosage of medication: 200 mg per tablet
d. Form of medication: 100 tablets
e. Expiration date:
f. Lot number or batch number:
g. Manufacturer: SmithKline Beecham Pharmaceuticals

Exercise 4.4 **Identifying the Components of Drug Labels**
(See page 106 for answers)

1.

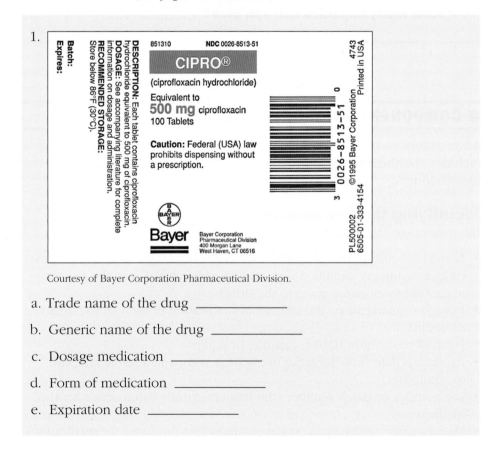

851310   NDC 0026-8513-51

CIPRO®

(ciprofloxacin hydrochloride)

Equivalent to
500 mg ciprofloxacin
100 Tablets

Caution: Federal (USA) law
prohibits dispensing without
a prescription.

Bayer
Bayer Corporation
Pharmaceutical Division
400 Morgan Lane
West Haven, CT 06516

DESCRIPTION: Each tablet contains ciprofloxacin
hydrochloride equivalent to 500 mg of ciprofloxacin.
DOSAGE: See accompanying literature for complete
information on dosage and administration.
RECOMMENDED STORAGE:
Store below 86°F (30°C).

Batch:
Expires:

4743
©1995 Bayer Corporation   Printed in USA

3 0026-8513-51 0

PL500002
6505-01-333-4154

Courtesy of Bayer Corporation Pharmaceutical Division.

a. Trade name of the drug _____

b. Generic name of the drug _____

c. Dosage medication _____

d. Form of medication _____

e. Expiration date _____

Exercise 4.5 — Problems With Components of Drug Labels
(See page 106 for answers)

1. Order: methylphenidate 10 mg PO before breakfast and lunch for attention-deficit hyperactivity disorder (ADHD)

▶ **How many tablets will you give?** _____

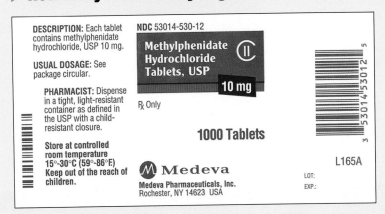

Courtesy of Medeva Pharmaceuticals.

2. Order: Xanax 500 mcg PO bid for anxiety

▶ **How many tablets will you give?** _____

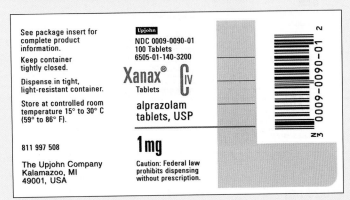

Courtesy of the Upjohn Company.

3. Order: Tolinase 375 mg PO every AM ac for type 2 diabetes mellitus

▶ **How many tablets will you give?** _____

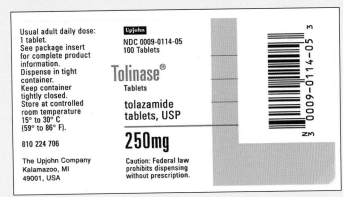

Courtesy of the Upjohn Company.

---

f. Batch number _____

g. Manufacturer _____

2.

Courtesy of SmithKline Beecham Pharmaceuticals.

a. Trade name of the drug _____

b. Generic name of the drug _____

c. Dosage medication _____

d. Form of medication _____

e. Expiration date _____

f. Batch number _____

g. Manufacturer _____

3.

Courtesy of the Upjohn Company.

a. Trade name of the drug _____

b. Generic name of the drug _____

c. Dosage medication _____

d. Form of medication _____

e. Expiration date _____

f. Batch number _____

g. Manufacturer _____

Solving Problems With Components of Drug Labels

Once you are able to identify the components of a drug label, you can use critical thinking to solve problems with dimensional analysis.

EXAMPLE 4.6

The physician orders Cipro 750 mg PO every 12 hours for a bacterial infection.

▶ **How many tablets will you give?**

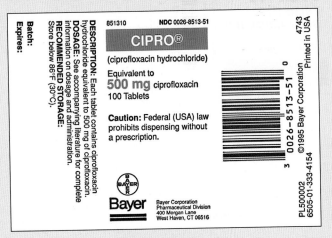

Courtesy of Bayer Corporation Pharmaceutical Division.

Given quantity   = 750 mg
Wanted quantity = tablets
Dose on hand   = 500 mg/tablet

Sequential method:

$$\frac{750 \text{ mg}}{} \left| \frac{\text{tablet}}{500 \text{ mg}} \right| \frac{75}{50} = 1.5 \text{ tablets}$$

▶▶▶ *1.5 tablets is the wanted quantity and the answer to the problem.*

EXAMPLE 4.7

Administer Tigan 200 mg PO qid for nausea.

▶ **How many capsules will you give?**

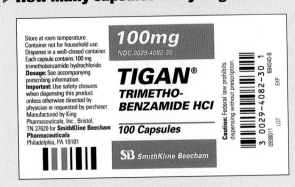

Courtesy of SmithKline Beecham Pharmaceuticals.

Given quantity   = 200 mg
Wanted quantity = capsules
Dose on hand   = 100 mg/capsules

Sequential method:

$$\frac{200 \text{ mg}}{} \left| \frac{\text{capsules}}{100 \text{ mg}} \right| \frac{2}{1} = 2 \text{ capsules}$$

▶▶▶ *2 capsules is the wanted quantity and the answer to the problem.*

EXAMPLE 4.8

Order: Halcion 0.25 mg PO at bedtime prn.

▶ **How many tablets will you give?**

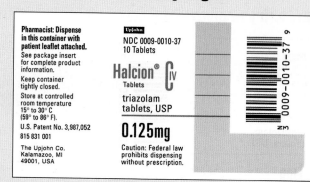

Courtesy of the Upjohn Company.

Given quantity   = 0.25 mg
Wanted quantity = tablets
Dose on hand   = 0.125 mg/tablet

Sequential method:

$$\frac{0.25 \text{ mg}}{} \left| \frac{\text{tablet}}{0.125 \text{ mg}} \right| \frac{0.25}{0.125} = 2 \text{ tablets}$$

▶▶▶ *2 tablets is the wanted quantity and the answer to the problem.*

4. Order: vitamin B$_{12}$ 2.5 mg daily as a daily vitamin supplement

▶ **How many tablets will you give?** _____

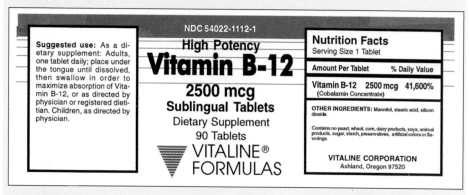

Courtesy of Vitaline Corporation.

5. Order: Tigan 250 mg PO qid prn for nausea

▶ **How many capsules will you give?** _____

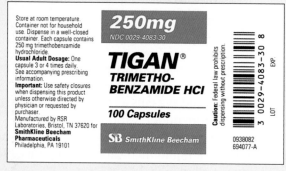

Courtesy of SmithKline Beecham Pharmaceuticals.

■ ADMINISTERING MEDICATION
   BY DIFFERENT ROUTES

Medication may be administered by various routes, including oral, parenteral, or intravenous, involving tablets, capsules, or liquid.

Enteral Medications

Oral (PO) medications are administered using tablets, caplets, capsules, or liquid. Tablets and caplets may be scored, which permits a more accurate administration when one fourth or one half of a tablet must be given.

Tablets and caplets may also be enteric coated, which allows the medication to bypass disintegration in the stomach to decrease irritation, and then later break down in the small intestine for absorption. Enteric-coated tablets and caplets should never be crushed, because such medications irritate the stomach.

PREVENTING MEDICATION ERRORS

Crushing enteric-coated tablets and caplets would be considered a **medication error** because the nurse did not administer the medication using the **right route.** The patient could suffer erosion of the esophagus or stomach resulting in a bleeding ulcer.

(Preventing Medication Errors continues on page 82)

Aspirin is an example of a medication that is enteric-coated to prevent erosion of gastrointestinal tissue.

PREVENTING MEDICATION ERRORS

Opening capsules and adding the medication to applesauce or pudding would also be considered a **medication error** because the nurse did not administer the medication using the **right route.** The patient could receive an incorrect dosage of the medication as the medication quickly enters the gastrointestinal system.

Capsules are usually of the time-release type, and these should never be crushed or opened because the medication would be immediately released into the system, instead of being released slowly over time.

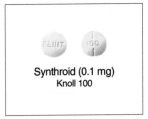

Synthroid (0.1 mg)
Knoll 100

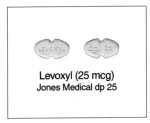

Levoxyl (25 mcg)
Jones Medical dp 25

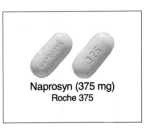

Naprosyn (375 mg)
Roche 375

Tablets: note scored tablet on right.

Caplets: note scored caplet on right.

Enteric-coated caplets.

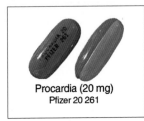

Procardia (20 mg)
Pfizer 20 261

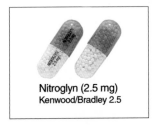

Nitroglyn (2.5 mg)
Kenwood/Bradley 2.5

Capsules.

Controlled-release capsules.

Liquid medication is accurately administered using a medication cup or medication syringe. The medication cup contains the common equivalents for the metric, apothecary, and household systems to permit adaptation of the medication's dosage for administration under various circumstances. The medication syringe contains the common equivalents for the metric and household systems to allow administration of liquid medications to infants, elderly, or anyone experiencing difficulty swallowing.

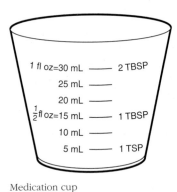

```
1 fl oz=30 mL ——— 2 TBSP
      25 mL ———
      20 mL ———
½ fl oz=15 mL ——— 1 TBSP
      10 mL ———
       5 mL ——— 1 TSP
```

Medication cup

Medication syringe

EXAMPLE 4.9

Order: Tagamet 600 mg PO bid for gastrointestinal (GI) bleeding.

▶ **How many tsp will you give?** _____

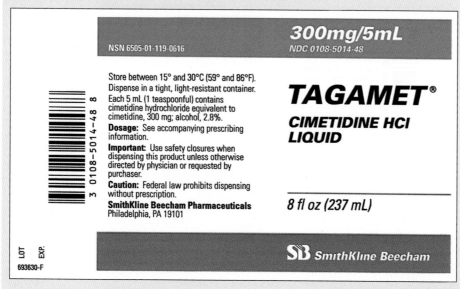

Courtesy of SmithKline Beecham Pharmaceuticals.

Given quantity   = 600 mg
Wanted quantity = tsp
Dose on hand   = 300 mg/5 mL

Sequential method:

$$\frac{600 \text{ mg}}{} \quad \frac{5 \text{ mL}}{300 \text{ mg}} \quad \frac{\text{tsp}}{5 \text{ mL}} \quad \frac{6 \times 5}{3 \times 5} \quad \frac{30}{15} = 2 \text{ tsp}$$

▶▶▶ *2 tsp is the wanted quantity and the answer to the problem.*

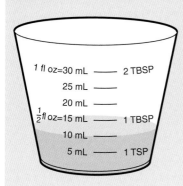

EXAMPLE 4.10

Order: Compazine 10 mg PO qid for psychomotor agitation.

▶ **How many mL will you give?** _____

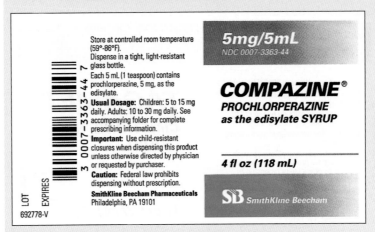

Courtesy of SmithKline Beecham Pharmaceuticals.

Given quantity   = 10 mg
Wanted quantity = mL
Dose on hand   = 5 mg/5 mL

Sequential method:

$$\frac{10 \text{ mg}}{} \;\bigg|\; \frac{5 \text{ mL}}{5 \text{ mg}} \;\bigg|\; \frac{10}{} = 10 \text{ mL}$$

▶▶▶ *10 mL is the wanted quantity and the answer to the problem.*

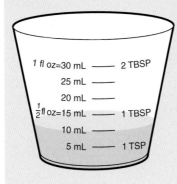

EXAMPLE 4.11

Order: Tegretol 100 mg PO qid for convulsions.

▶ **How many tsp will you give?** _____

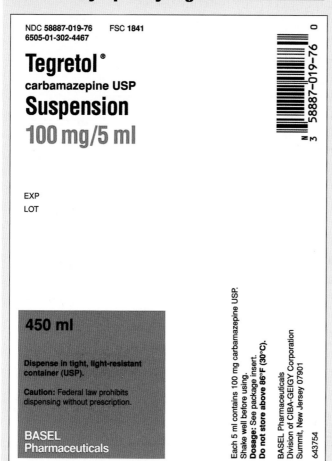

NDC 58887-019-76   FSC 1841
6505-01-302-4467

Tegretol®
carbamazepine USP
Suspension
100 mg/5 ml

N 3 58887-019-76 0

EXP
LOT

450 ml

Dispense in tight, light-resistant container (USP).

Caution: Federal law prohibits dispensing without prescription.

BASEL
Pharmaceuticals

Each 5 ml contains 100 mg carbamazepine USP.
Shake well before using.
Dosage: See package insert.
Do not store above 86°F (30°C).

BASEL Pharmaceuticals
Division of CIBA-GEIGY Corporation
Summit, New Jersey 07901

643754

Courtesy of Basel Pharmaceuticals.

Given quantity   = 100 mg
Wanted quantity = tsp
Dose on hand   = 100 mg/5 mL

Random method:

$$\frac{\cancel{100\ mg}}{} \cdot \frac{1\ \text{tsp}}{5\ \cancel{mL}} \cdot \frac{5\ \cancel{mL}}{\cancel{100\ mg}} \cdot \frac{1}{} = 1\ tsp$$

▶▶▶ *1 tsp is the wanted quantity and the answer to the problem.*

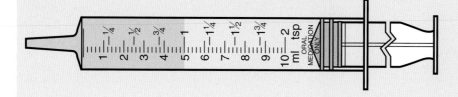

Exercise 4.6 **Administering Enteral Medications**
(See pages 106–107 for answers)

1. Order: phenobarbital gr $\frac{1}{2}$ PO daily for convulsions

   On hand: 20 mg/5 mL

   ▶ **How many mL will you give?** _____

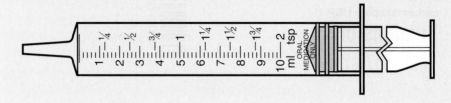

2. Order: Zantac 0.15 g PO bid for ulcers

   On hand: 15 mg/mL

   ▶ **How many tsp will you give?** _____

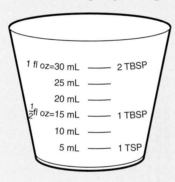

3. Order: Dilaudid 3 mg PO every 3 hours prn for pain

   On hand: Dilaudid Liquid 1 mg/mL

   ▶ **How many mL will you give?** _____

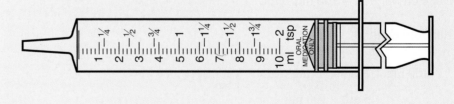

4. Order: lactulose 20 g PO tid for hepatic encephalopathy

On hand: lactulose 10 g/15 mL

▶ **How many oz will you give?** _____

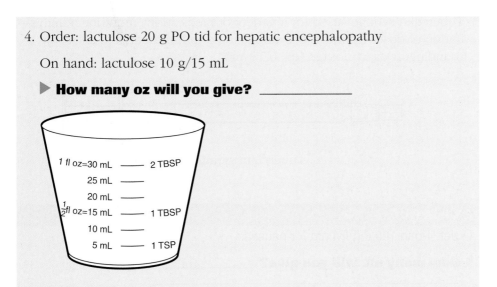

Parenteral Medications

Medications may also be ordered by the physician for the parenteral route of administration, including subcutaneous (SQ), intramuscular (IM), and intravenous (IV). Parenteral medications are sterile solutions obtained from vials or ampules and are administered using a syringe or prefilled syringes. The three syringes most often used are:

1. 3-mL syringe (used for a variety of medications requiring administration of doses from 0.2 to 3 mL).

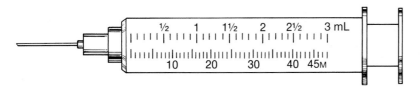

3-mL syringe

2. Insulin syringe (used specifically to administer insulin). Two types are illustrated below **A.** 0.5-mL low-dose syringe for U-100 insulin and **B.** 1-mL syringe for U-100 insulin.

A

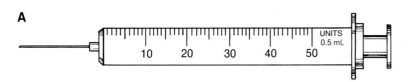

0.5-mL low-dose syringe

B

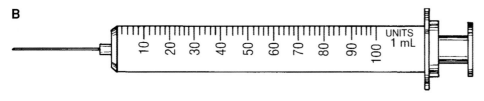

1-mL syringe

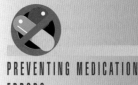

PREVENTING MEDICATION ERRORS

It is the responsibility of the nurse to choose the correct syringe when administering parenteral medications. The nurse can prevent **medication errors** by being knowledgeable about different types of syringes and when it is appropriate to use specific syringes.

Insulin is manufactured in different strengths and a variety of types based on onset, peak, and duration. Lilly and Novo Nordisk are the primary providers of insulin. Insulin is classified as rapid acting (Humalog and Novolog), short-acting (Regular Insulin), intermediate (NPH and Lente), and long-acting (Lantus, and Ultralente). Some types of insulin must be administered in a single syringe, and other types of insulin can be mixed in a single syringe for administration.

Insulin is given with an insulin syringe that requires no calculation. The number of units of insulin ordered by the physician equals the number of units that the nurse draws using the correct insulin syringe: low-dose or regular U-100.

It is the responsibility of the nurse to be familiar with the different types of insulin and to use a nursing drug reference to prevent medication errors associated with insulin administration. Every nurse should know the onset, peak, and duration of the insulin being administered as well as

(Preventing Medication Errors continues on page 88)

the signs and symptoms of hypoglycemia (pale, cool, clammy skin and hunger) and hyperglycemia (hot, red, dry skin and thirst).

PREVENTING MEDICATION ERRORS

The nurse needs to be familiar with the different types of anticoagulants (heparin, Warfarin, and Coumadin) to ensure patient safety and prevent **medication errors.** The nurse needs to know which laboratory value to monitor (PT, PTT, INR) and which antidote (protamine sulfate or vitamin K) to have available for emergencies.

Heparin is an anticoagulant that is used to decrease the clotting ability of the blood and help prevent harmful clots from forming in the blood vessels. Although heparin is commonly referred to as a blood thinner, it does not dissolve blood clots that have already formed. Heparin may help prevent blood clots from becoming larger and causing more serious problems to the heart or lungs.

Heparin is administered using a tuberculin syringe, which is calibrated from 0.1 to 1 mL. This allows for more accurate administration of medication dosages of less than 1 mL.

3. Tuberculin syringe (used for a variety of medications requiring administration of doses from 0.1 to 1 mL). Marked in hundredths to allow for rounding or exact dosage (eg, 0.75 mL).

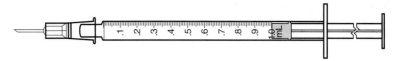

Tuberculin syringe

EXAMPLE 4.12

Order: Tigan 100 mg IM qid for nausea.

▶ **How many mL will you give?** _____

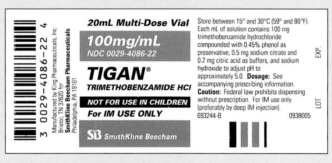

Courtesy of SmithKline Beecham Pharmaceuticals.

Given quantity   = 100 mg
Wanted quantity = mL
Dose on hand   = 100 mg/mL

Sequential method:

$$\frac{100 \text{ mg}}{} \cdot \frac{\text{mL}}{100 \text{ mg}} \cdot \frac{1}{1} = 1 \text{ mL}$$

▶▶▶ *1 mL is the wanted quantity and the answer to the problem.*

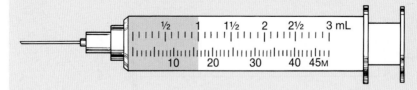

EXAMPLE 4.13

Order: Compazine 10 mg IM every 4 hours for psychoses.

▶ **How many mL will you give?** _____

Store below 86°F. Do not freeze.
Protect from light. Discard if markedly discolored.
Each mL contains, in aqueous solution, prochlorper-
azine, 5 mg, as the edisylate; sodium biphosphate,
5 mg; sodium tartrate, 12 mg; sodium saccharin,
0.9 mg; benzyl alcohol, 0.75%, as preservative.
Dosage: For deep I.M. or I.V. injection.
See accompanying prescribing information.
Caution: Federal law prohibits dispensing without
prescription.
SmithKline Beecham Pharmaceuticals
LOT   EXP.
693793-AD Philadelphia, PA 19101

10mL Multi-Dose Vial
5mg/mL
NDC 0007-3343-01
COMPAZINE®
PROCHLORPERAZINE
as the edisylate INJECTION
SB SmithKline Beecham

Courtesy of SmithKline Beecham Pharmaceuticals.

Given quantity   = 10 mg
Wanted quantity = mL
Dose on hand   = 5 mg/mL

Sequential method:

$$\frac{10 \text{ mg}}{} \left| \frac{\text{mL}}{5 \text{ mg}} \right| \frac{10}{5} = 2 \text{ mL}$$

▶▶▶ *2 mL is the wanted quantity and the answer to the problem.*

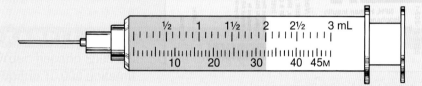

EXAMPLE 4.14

Order: morphine sulfate, $\frac{1}{4}$ gr every 4 hours prn for pain.

▶ **How many mL will you give?** _____

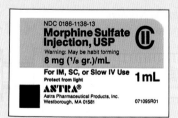

NDC 0186-1138-13
Morphine Sulfate Ⓒ
Injection, USP
Warning: May be habit forming
8 mg (¹/₈ gr.)/mL
For IM, SC, or Slow IV Use   **1 mL**
Protect from light
ASTRA®
Astra Pharmaceutical Products, Inc.
Westborough, MA 01581   071095R01

Courtesy of Astra Pharmaceutical Products.

Given quantity   = $\frac{1}{4}$ gr
Wanted quantity = mL
Dose on hand   = 8 mg/mL or $\frac{1}{8}$ gr/mL

(Example continues on page 90)

Summary

This chapter has taught you to interpret medication orders and drug labels and to calculate one-factor medication problems using dimensional analysis. To demonstrate your ability to interpret correctly and calculate accurately, complete the following practice problems.

Practice Problems for Chapter 4	One-Factor Medication Problems

One-Factor Medication Problems
(See pages 107–108 for answers)

1. The physician orders Tigan 0.2 g IM qid for nausea. The dosage of medication on hand is a multiple-dose vial labeled 100 mg/mL.

   ▶ **How many mL will you give?** _____

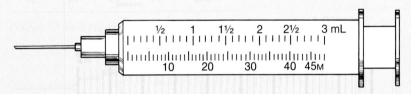

2. A physician orders Thorazine 50 mg tid prn for singultus. The dose on hand is Thorazine 25-mg tablets.

   ▶ **How many tablets will you give?** _____

3. Order: Orinase 1 g PO bid for type 2 diabetes mellitus

   ▶ **How many tablets will you give?** _____

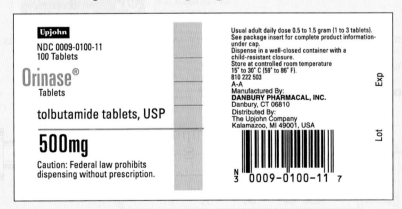

Courtesy of the Upjohn Company.

4. Order: Persantine 50 mg PO qid for prevention of thromboembolism

▶ **How many tablets will you give?** _____

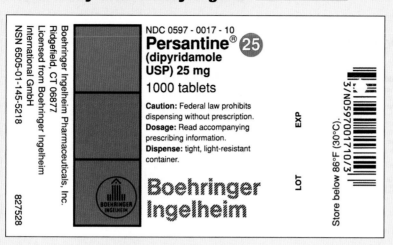

Courtesy of Boehringer Ingelheim Pharmaceuticals.

5. Order: NPH insulin 56 units SQ every AM for type 1 diabetes mellitus

On hand: NPH insulin 100 units/mL

▶ **How many units will you give?** _____

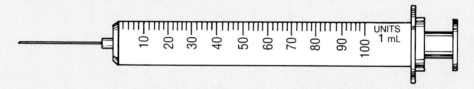

6. Order: heparin 7500 units SQ bid for prevention of thrombi

On hand: heparin 10,000 units/mL

▶ **How many mL will you give?** _____

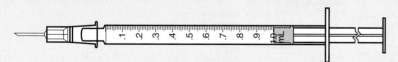

(Practice Problems continue on page 96)

7. Order: Augmentin 500 mg PO every 8 hours for infection.

▶ **How many mL will you give?** _____

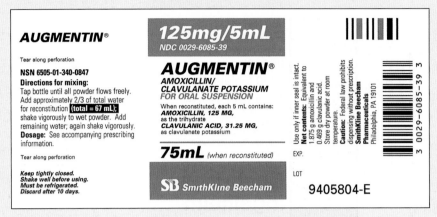

Courtesy of SmithKline Beecham Pharmaceuticals.

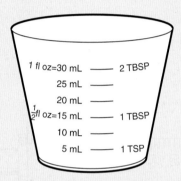

8. Order: Zaroxolyn 5 mg PO every AM for hypertension

▶ **How many tablets will you give?** _____

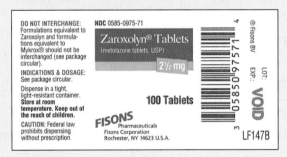

Courtesy of Fisons Pharmaceuticals.

9. Order: methylphenidate (Ritalin) 10 mg PO tid for attention-deficit
hyperactivity disorder (ADHD)

   ▶ **How many tablets will you give?** _____

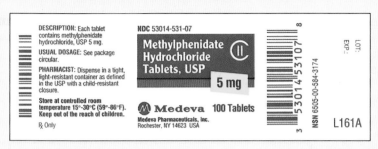

   Courtesy of Medeva Pharmaceuticals.

10. Order: meperidine 50 mg IM every 3 hours prn for pain.

    On hand: meperidine 100 mg/mL

    ▶ **How many mL will you give?** _____

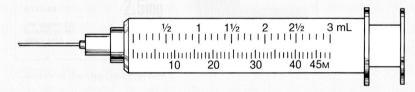

7. Order: hydromorphone 3 mg IM every 3 hours for pain

▶ **How many milliliters will you give?** _____

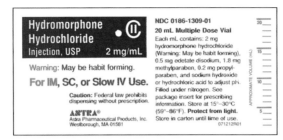

Courtesy of Astra Pharmaceutical Products.

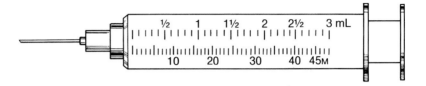

8. Order: magnesium sulfate 1000 mg IM in each buttock for

hypomagnesemia

▶ **How many milliliters will you give?** _____

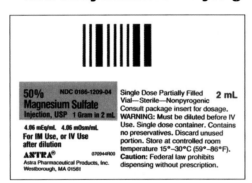

Courtesy of Astra Pharmaceutical Products.

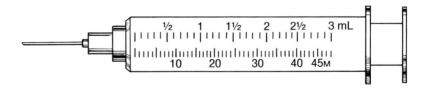

9. Order: naloxone HCl 200 mcg IV stat for respiratory depression

▶ **How many milliliters will you give?** _____

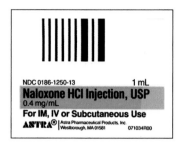

Courtesy of Astra Pharmaceutical
Products.

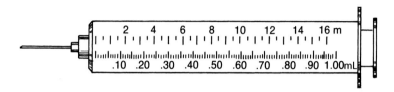

10. Order: Solu-Medrol 40 mg IM daily for autoimmune disorder

▶ **How many milliliters will you give?** _____

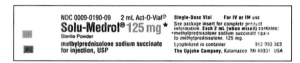

Courtesy of the Upjohn Company.

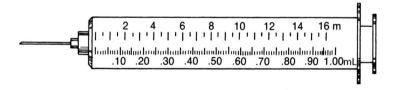

ANSWER KEY FOR CHAPTER 4: ONE-FACTOR MEDICATION PROBLEMS

Exercise 4.1 Interpretation of Medication Orders

1

a. Right patient   Mrs. A. Clark
b. Right drug   Aspirin for fever
c. Right dosage   gr 10
d. Right route   orally (PO)
e. Right time   every 4 hr as needed (prn)
f. Right documentation: The patient's name, the drug, the dosage, the route administered and the date and time administered should be charted on the Medication Administration Record (MAR). Aspirin is a prn medication and therefore the reason the drug was administered and the effects following administration of the drug should also be charted on the MAR. The nurse's signature and initials should appear on the MAR.

2

a. Right patient   Mr. W. Smith
b. Right drug   Advil (ibuprofen) for arthritis
c. Right dosage   400 mg
d. Right route   PO (orally)
e. Right time   every 6 hr
f. Right documentation: The patient's name, the drug, the dosage, the route administered and the date and time administered should be charted on the Medication Administration Record (MAR). Advil is a regularly scheduled medication and the reason for the drug administration is listed as arthritis. The nurse's signature and initials should appear on the MAR.

3

a. Right patient   Mr. T. Jones
b. Right drug   Tylenol (acetaminophen) for headache
c. Right dosage   gr 10
d. Right route   PO (orally)
e. Right time   every 4 hr prn
f. Right documentation: The patient's name, the drug, the dosage, the route administered and the date and time administered should be charted on the Medication Administration Record (MAR). Tylenol is a prn medication and therefore the reason the drug was administered and the effects following administration of the drug should also be charted. The nurse's signature and initials should appear on the MAR.

Exercise 4.3 One-Factor Medication Problems

1. Sequential method:

$$\frac{0.25\ \text{g}}{}\left|\frac{1000\ \text{mg}}{1\ \text{g}}\right|\frac{\text{capsule}}{250\ \text{mg}}\left|\frac{0.25 \times 100}{1 \times 25}\right|\frac{25}{25} = 1\ \text{capsule}$$

Random method:

$$\frac{0.25\ \text{g}}{}\left|\frac{\text{capsule}}{250\ \text{mg}}\right|\frac{1000\ \text{mg}}{1\ \text{g}}\left|\frac{0.25 \times 100}{25 \times 1}\right|\frac{25}{25} = 1\ \text{capsule}$$

2. Sequential method:

$$\frac{\frac{1}{2}\ \text{gr}}{}\left|\frac{60\ \text{mg}}{1\ \text{gr}}\right|\frac{\text{tablet}}{15\ \text{mg}}\left|\frac{\frac{1}{2} \times \frac{60}{1}}{1 \times 15}\right|\frac{\frac{60}{2}}{15}\left|\frac{30}{15}\right. = 2\ \text{tablets}$$

Random method:

$$\frac{\frac{1}{2}\ \text{gr}}{}\left|\frac{\text{tablet}}{15\ \text{mg}}\right|\frac{60\ \text{mg}}{1\ \text{gr}}\left|\frac{\frac{1}{2} \times \frac{60}{1}}{15 \times 1}\right|\frac{\frac{60}{2}}{15}\left|\frac{30}{15}\right. = 2\ \text{tablets}$$

3. Sequential method:

$$\frac{0.5\ \text{g}}{}\left|\frac{1000\ \text{mg}}{1\ \text{g}}\right|\frac{\text{tablet}}{500\ \text{mg}}\left|\frac{0.5 \times 10}{1 \times 5}\right|\frac{5}{5} = 1\ \text{tablet}$$

Random method:

$$\frac{0.5\ \text{g}}{}\left|\frac{\text{tablet}}{500\ \text{mg}}\right|\frac{1000\ \text{mg}}{1\ \text{g}}\left|\frac{0.5 \times 10}{5 \times 1}\right|\frac{5}{5} = 1\ \text{tablet}$$

4. Sequential method:

$$\frac{0.03\ \text{g}}{}\left|\frac{1000\ \text{mg}}{1\ \text{g}}\right|\frac{\text{capsules}}{30\ \text{mg}}\left|\frac{0.03 \times 100}{1 \times 3}\right|\frac{3}{3} = 1\ \text{capsule}$$

Random method:

$$\frac{0.03\ \text{g}}{}\left|\frac{\text{capsules}}{30\ \text{mg}}\right|\frac{1000\ \text{mg}}{1\ \text{g}}\left|\frac{0.03 \times 100}{3 \times 1}\right|\frac{3}{3} = 1\ \text{capsule}$$

5. Sequential method:

$$\frac{\frac{1}{2}\ \text{gr}}{}\bigg|\frac{60\ \text{mg}}{1\ \text{gr}}\bigg|\frac{\boxed{\text{capsules}}}{30\ \text{mg}}\bigg|\frac{\frac{1}{2}\times\frac{60}{1}}{1\times30}\bigg|\frac{\frac{60}{2}}{30}\bigg|\frac{30}{30}=1\ \text{capsule}$$

Random method:

$$\frac{\frac{1}{2}\ \text{gr}}{}\bigg|\frac{\boxed{\text{capsules}}}{30\ \text{mg}}\bigg|\frac{60\ \text{mg}}{1\ \text{gr}}\bigg|\frac{\frac{1}{2}\times\frac{60}{1}}{30\times1}\bigg|\frac{\frac{60}{2}}{30}\bigg|\frac{30}{30}=1\ \text{capsule}$$

Exercise 4.4 Identifying the Components of Drug Labels

1
a. Cipro
b. Ciprofloxacin hydrochloride
c. 500 mg per tablet
d. 100 tablets
e. *Not listed on the label
f. *Not listed on the label
g. Bayer Corporation, Pharmaceutical Division

2
a. Tigan
b. Trimethobenzamide hydrochloride
c. 100 mg per capsule
d. 100 capsules
e. *Not listed on the label
f. *Not listed on the label
g. SmithKline Beecham Pharmaceuticals

3
a. Halcion
b. Triazolam
c. 0.125 mg per tablet
d. 10 tablets
e. *Not listed on the label
f. *Not listed on the label
g. The Upjohn Company

Exercise 4.5 Problems With Components of Drug Labels

1. Sequential method:

$$\frac{10\ \text{mg}}{}\bigg|\frac{\boxed{\text{tablet}}}{10\ \text{mg}}\bigg|\frac{10}{10}=1\ \text{tablet}$$

2. Random method:

$$\frac{500\ \text{mcg}}{}\bigg|\frac{\boxed{\text{tablet}}}{1\ \text{mg}}\bigg|\frac{1\ \text{mg}}{1000\ \text{mcg}}\bigg|\frac{5}{10}=\frac{1}{2}\ \text{tablet}$$

3. Sequential method:

$$\frac{375\ \text{mg}}{}\bigg|\frac{\boxed{\text{tablet}}}{250\ \text{mg}}\bigg|\frac{375}{250}=1\tfrac{1}{2}\ \text{tablets}$$

4. Random method:

$$\frac{2.5\ \text{mg}}{}\bigg|\frac{\boxed{\text{tablet}}}{2500\ \text{mcg}}\bigg|\frac{1000\ \text{mcg}}{1\ \text{mg}}\bigg|\frac{2.5\times10}{25\times1}\bigg|\frac{25}{25}=1\ \text{tablet}$$

5. Sequential method:

$$\frac{250\ \text{mg}}{}\bigg|\frac{\boxed{\text{capsule}}}{250\ \text{mg}}\bigg|\frac{25}{25}=1\ \text{capsule}$$

Exercise 4.6 Administering Enteral Medications

1. Random method:

$$\frac{\frac{1}{2}\ \text{gr}}{}\bigg|\frac{5\ \boxed{\text{mL}}}{20\ \text{mg}}\bigg|\frac{60\ \text{mg}}{1\ \text{gr}}\bigg|\frac{\frac{1}{2}\times\frac{5}{1}\times\frac{6}{1}}{2\times1}\bigg|\frac{\frac{30}{2}}{2}\bigg|\frac{15}{2}=7.5\ \text{mL}$$

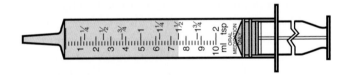

2. Sequential method:

$$\frac{0.15\ \text{g}}{}\bigg|\frac{1000\ \text{mg}}{1\ \text{g}}\bigg|\frac{\text{mL}}{15\ \text{mg}}\bigg|\frac{1\ \boxed{\text{tsp}}}{5\ \text{mL}}\bigg|\frac{0.15\times1000}{15\times5}\bigg|\frac{150}{75}=2\ \text{tsp}$$

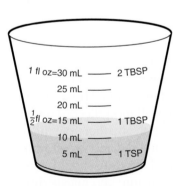

3. Sequential method:

$$\frac{3 \text{ mg}}{} \left| \frac{\text{mL}}{1 \text{ mg}} \right| \frac{3}{1} = 3 \text{ mL}$$

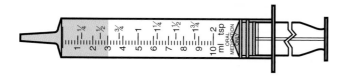

4. Sequential method:

$$\frac{20 \text{ g}}{} \left| \frac{15 \text{ mL}}{10 \text{ g}} \right| \frac{1 \text{ oz}}{30 \text{ mL}} \left| \frac{2 \times 15 \times 1}{1 \times 30} \right| \frac{30}{30} = 1 \text{ oz}$$

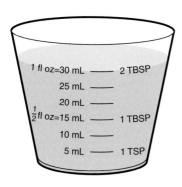

Exercise 4.7 Administering Parenteral Medications

1. Random method:

$$\frac{300 \text{ mcg}}{} \left| \frac{\text{mL}}{0.1 \text{ mg}} \right| \frac{1 \text{ mg}}{1000 \text{ mcg}} \left| \frac{3 \times 1}{0.1 \times 10} \right| \frac{3}{1} = 3 \text{ mL}$$

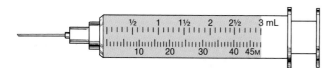

2. Sequential method:

$$\frac{3 \text{ mg}}{} \left| \frac{\text{mL}}{2 \text{ mg}} \right| \frac{3}{2} = 1.5 \text{ mL}$$

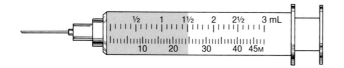

3. Sequential method:

$$\frac{35 \text{ mg}}{} \left| \frac{\text{mL}}{10 \text{ mg}} \right| \frac{35}{10} = 3.5 \text{ mL}$$

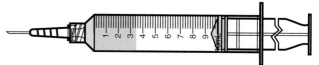

4. Sequential method:

$$\frac{10 \text{ units}}{} \left| \right. = 10 \text{ units}$$

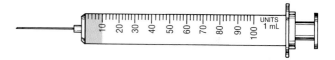

5. Sequential method:

$$\frac{8000 \text{ units}}{} \left| \frac{\text{mL}}{10,000 \text{ units}} \right| \frac{8}{10} = 0.8 \text{ mL}$$

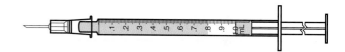

Practice Problems

1. Random method:

$$\frac{0.2 \text{ g}}{} \left| \frac{\text{mL}}{100 \text{ mg}} \right| \frac{1000 \text{ mg}}{1 \text{ g}} \left| \frac{0.2 \times 10}{1 \times 1} \right| \frac{2}{1} = 2 \text{ mL}$$

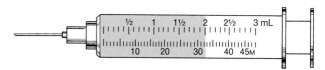

2. Sequential method:

$$\frac{50 \text{ mg}}{} \left| \frac{\text{tablet}}{25 \text{ mg}} \right| \frac{50}{25} = 2 \text{ tablets}$$

3. Random method:

$$\frac{1\text{ g}}{500\text{ mg}}\Bigg|\frac{\text{(tablet)}}{}\Bigg|\frac{1000\text{ mg}}{1\text{ g}}\Bigg|\frac{1\times10}{5\times1}\Bigg|\frac{10}{5}=2\text{ tablets}$$

4. Random method:

$$\frac{50\text{ mg}}{25\text{ mg}}\Bigg|\frac{\text{(tablet)}}{}\Bigg|\frac{50}{25}=2\text{ tablets}$$

5. Sequential method:

$$\frac{56\text{ units}}{}\Bigg|\frac{}{}=56\text{ units}$$

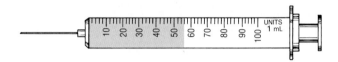

6. Sequential method:

$$\frac{7500\text{ units}}{}\Bigg|\frac{\text{(mL)}}{10000\text{ units}}\Bigg|\frac{75}{100}=0.75\text{ mL}$$

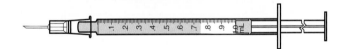

7. Sequential method:

$$\frac{500\text{ mg}}{}\Bigg|\frac{5\text{ (mL)}}{125\text{ mg}}\Bigg|\frac{500\times5}{125}\Bigg|\frac{2500}{125}=20\text{ mL}$$

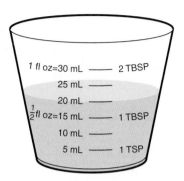

8. Sequential method:

$$\frac{5\text{ mg}}{2.5\text{ mg}}\Bigg|\frac{\text{(tablet)}}{}\Bigg|\frac{5}{2.5}=2\text{ tablets}$$

9. Sequential method:

$$\frac{10\text{ mg}}{5\text{ mg}}\Bigg|\frac{\text{(tablet)}}{}\Bigg|\frac{10}{5}=2\text{ tablets}$$

10. Sequential method:

$$\frac{50\text{ mg}}{100\text{ mg}}\Bigg|\frac{\text{(mL)}}{10}\Bigg|\frac{5}{10}=0.5\text{ mL}$$

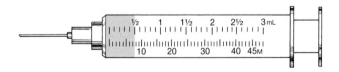

CHAPTER 5

Two-Factor Medication Problems

Objectives

After completing this chapter, you will successfully be able to:

1. Solve two-factor–given quantity to one-factor–wanted quantity medication problems involving a specific amount of medication ordered based on the weight of the patient.
2. Calculate medication problems requiring reconstitution of medications by using information from a nursing drug reference, label, or package insert.
3. Solve two-factor–given quantity to two-factor–wanted quantity medication problems involving a specific amount of fluid to be delivered over limited time using an intravenous pump delivering milliliters per hour (mL/hr).
4. Solve two-factor–given quantity to two-factor–wanted quantity medication problems involving a specific amount of fluid to be delivered over a limited time using different types of intravenous tubing that deliver drops per minute (gtt/min) based on a specific drop factor.

Outline

Although medications are ordered by physicians or nurse practitioners and administered by nurses using the "six rights of medication administration," other factors must be considered when administering certain medications or intravenous (IV) fluids.

PREVENTING MEDICATION ERRORS

The **weight** of the patient often must be factored into a medication problem when determining how much medication can safely be given to an infant or a child or an elderly patient.

The dosage of medication available may be in a powdered form that needs **reconstitution** to a liquid form before parenteral or IV administration.

Also, the length of **time** over which medication or IV fluids can be given plays an important role in the safe administration of IV therapy.

To be able to calculate a two-factor–given quantity to one-factor– or two-factor–wanted quantity medication problem, it is important to understand all factors that may need to be considered in some medication problems. With use of dimensional analysis, this chapter will teach you to calculate medication problems involving the weight of the patient, the reconstitution of medications from powder to liquid form, and the amount of time over which medications or IV fluids can be safely administered.

■ MEDICATION PROBLEMS INVOLVING WEIGHT

When solving problems with dimensional analysis, you can use either the *sequential method* or the *random method* to calculate two-factor–given quantity medication problems. The **given quantity** (the physician's order) contains two parts including a **numerator** (dosage of medication) and a **denominator** (the weight of the patient). This type of medication problem is called a *two-factor* medication problem because the *given quantity* now contains two parts (a numerator and a denominator) instead of just one part (a numerator).

Below is an example of the problem-solving method showing placement of basic terms used in dimensional analysis, applied to a two-factor medication problem involving weight.

Unit Path

Given Quantity	Conversion Factor for Given Quantity (Numerator)		Conversion Factor for Given Quantity (Denominator)		Conversion Computation		Wanted Quantity
2.5 mg	mL		1 kg	60 lb	$2.5 \times 1 \times 6$	15	$= 1.7$ mL
kg	40 mg		2.2 lb		4.22	8.8	

THINKING IT THROUGH

The two-factor–given quantity has been set up with a numerator (2.5 mg) and a denominator (kg) leading across the unit path to a one-factor–wanted quantity with only a numerator (mL).

The *dose on hand* (40 mg/mL) has been factored in to cancel out the preceding unwanted unit (mg). The wanted unit (mL) is in the numerator and corresponds with the one-factor–wanted quantity (mL).

EXAMPLE 5.1

The physician orders gentamicin 2.5 mg/kg IV (intravenous) every 8 hours for infection. The vial of medication is labeled 40 mg/mL. The child weighs 60 lb.

▶ **How many milliliters will you give?** _____

Given quantity   = 2.5 mg/kg
Wanted quantity = mL
Dose on hand   = 40 mg/mL
Weight   = 60 lb

Sequential method:

STEP 1 Identify the two-factor–given quantity (the physician's order).

Unit Path

Given Quantity	Conversion Factor for Given Quantity (Numerator)	Conversion Factor for Given Quantity (Denominator)	Conversion Computation	Wanted Quantity
2.5 mg				
kg				= mL

STEP 2

Unit Path

Given Quantity	Conversion Factor for Given Quantity (Numerator)	Conversion Factor for Given Quantity (Denominator)	Conversion Computation	Wanted Quantity
2.5 mg	(mL)			
kg	40 mg			= mL

STEP 3

Unit Path

Given Quantity	Conversion Factor for Given Quantity (Numerator)	Conversion Factor for Given Quantity (Denominator)	Conversion Computation	Wanted Quantity
2.5 ~~mg~~	(mL)	1 ~~kg~~		
~~kg~~	40 ~~mg~~	2.2 lb		= mL

STEP 4

Unit Path

Given Quantity	Conversion Factor for Given Quantity (Numerator)	Conversion Factor for Given Quantity (Denominator)	Conversion Computation	Wanted Quantity
2.5 ~~mg~~	(mL)	1 ~~kg~~	60 ~~lb~~	
~~kg~~	40 ~~mg~~	2.2 ~~lb~~		= mL

(Example continues on page 112)

A *conversion factor* (1 kg = 2.2 lb) is factored into the unit path to cancel out the preceding unwanted unit (kg).

The *weight* is finally factored in to cancel out the preceding unwanted unit (lb) in the denominator. All unwanted units are canceled and only the wanted unit (mL) remains and corresponds with the wanted quantity (mL). Multiply the numerators, multiply the denominators, and divide the product of the numerators by the product of the denominators to provide the numerical value.

PREVENTING MEDICATION ERRORS

One of the most frequent **medication errors** is the error made with the conversion of weight.

The weight conversion [1 kg = 2.2 lb] is often incorrectly written [1 lb = 2.2 kg].

Remember that you would rather tell someone your weight in kilograms as it is a much smaller number [1 kg = 2.2 lb or, put in more realistic terms, 90.9 kg = 200 lb].

STEP 5

Unit Path

Given Quantity	Conversion Factor for Given Quantity (Numerator)	Conversion Factor for Given Quantity (Denominator)	Conversion Computation		Wanted Quantity
2.5 ~~mg~~	(mL)	1 ~~kg~~	60 ~~lb~~	$2.5 \times 1 \times 6$	15	$= 1.7$ mL
~~kg~~	40 ~~mg~~	2.2 ~~lb~~		4×2.2	8.8	

▶ ▶ ▶ *1.7 mL is the wanted quantity and the answer to the problem.*

Dimensional analysis is a problem-solving method that uses critical thinking. When implementing the *random method* of dimensional analysis, the medication problem can be set up in a number of different ways. The focus is on the correct placement of conversion factors to cancel out all unwanted units. The wanted unit is placed in the numerator to correctly correspond with the wanted quantity.

$$\frac{2.5 \text{ mg} \mid 1 \text{ kg} \mid 60 \text{ lb} \mid \text{mL} \mid 2.5 \times 1 \times 6 \mid 15}{\text{kg} \mid 2.2 \text{ lb} \mid \mid 40 \text{ mg} \mid 2.2 \times 4 \mid 8.8} = 1.7 \text{ mL}$$

Exercise 5.1	**Pediatric Medication Problems Involving Weight**
	(See page 137 for answers)

1. Order: furosemide 1 mg/kg IV bid for hypercalcemia. The child weighs 45 lb.

   ▶ **How many milliliters will you give?** _____

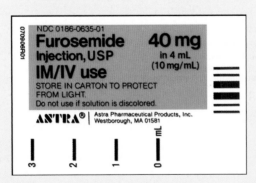

Courtesy of Astra Pharmaceutical Products.

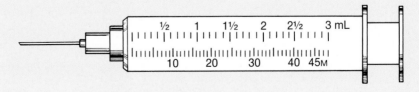

2. Order: atropine sulfate 0.01 mg/kg IV stat for bradycardia. The child weighs 20 lb.

▶ **How many milliliters will you give?** _____

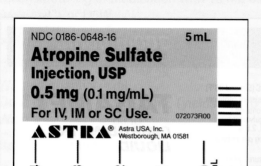

> NDC 0186-0648-16   5 mL
>
> **Atropine Sulfate**
> Injection, USP
> **0.5 mg** (0.1 mg/mL)
> For IV, IM or SC Use.   072073R00
>
> **ASTRA®** Astra USA, Inc.
>   Westborough, MA 01581

Courtesy of Astra Pharmaceutical Products.

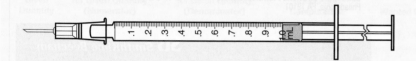

3. Order: phenergan 0.5 mg/kg IV every 4 hours prn for nausea. The dose on hand is 25 mg/mL. The child weighs 45 lb.

▶ **How many milliliters will you give?** _____

4. Order: morphine 50 mcg/kg IV every 4 hours prn for pain. The child weighs 75 lb.

▶ **How many milliliters will you give?** _____

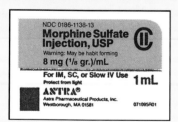

> NDC 0186-1138-13
> **Morphine Sulfate** **Ⓒ II**
> **Injection, USP**
> Warning: May be habit forming
> **8 mg** (¹/₈ gr.)/mL
>
> For IM, SC, or Slow IV Use
> Protect from light   **1 mL**
> **ASTRA®**
> Astra Pharmaceutical Products, Inc.
> Westborough, MA 01581   071095R01

Courtesy of Astra Pharmaceutical Products.

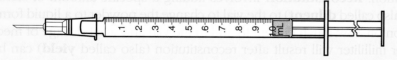

(Exercise continues on page 114)

Random method:

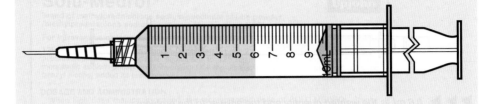

$$\frac{50 \text{ mg}}{\text{kg}} \left| \frac{10 \text{ mL}}{1 \text{ g}} \right| \frac{1 \text{ g}}{1000 \text{ mg}} \left| 12 \text{ kg} \right| \frac{5 \times 1 \times 1 \times 12}{1 \times 10} \left| \frac{60}{10} \right. = 6 \text{ mL}$$

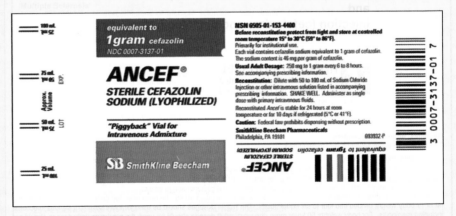

▶▶▶ *6 mL is the wanted quantity and the answer to the problem.*

Exercise 5.2   **Medication Problems Involving Reconstitution**
(See pages 137–138 for answers)

1. Order: Ancef 500 mg IV every 8 hours for infection.

   ▶ **How many milliliters will you draw out of the vial after reconstitution?** _____

   (Ancef is reconstituted using 50 mL sodium chloride.)

— 100 mL.	**equivalent to**	**NSN 6505-01-153-4400**
— 2 mL	**1 gram** cefazolin	Before reconstitution protect from light and store at controlled room temperature 15° to 30°C (59° to 86°F).
	NDC 0007-3137-01	Primarily for institutional use.

   Label reads:

   equivalent to 1 gram cefazolin
   NDC 0007-3137-01

   ANCEF®
   STERILE CEFAZOLIN
   SODIUM (LYOPHILIZED)

   "Piggyback" Vial for Intravenous Admixture

   SB SmithKline Beecham

   NSN 6505-01-153-4400
   Before reconstitution protect from light and store at controlled room temperature 15° to 30°C (59° to 86°F).
   Primarily for institutional use.
   Each vial contains cefazolin sodium equivalent to 1 gram of cefazolin. The sodium content is 46 mg per gram of cefazolin.
   Usual Adult Dosage: 250 mg to 1 gram every 6 to 8 hours. See accompanying prescribing information.
   Reconstitution: Dilute with 50 to 100 mL of Sodium Chloride Injection or other intravenous solution listed in accompanying prescribing information. SHAKE WELL. Administer as single dose with primary intravenous fluids.
   Reconstituted Ancef is stable for 24 hours at room temperature or for 10 days if refrigerated (5°C or 41°F).
   Caution: Federal law prohibits dispensing without prescription.
   SmithKline Beecham Pharmaceuticals
   Philadelphia, PA 19101   693932-P

   3 0007-3137-01 7

   Courtesy of SmithKline Beecham Pharmaceuticals.

2. Order: Primaxin 250 mg IV every 6 hours for infection

   Supply: Primaxin vial labeled 500 mg. Reconstitute with 10 mL of compatible diluent and shake well.

   ▶ **How many milliliters will you draw from the vial after reconstitution?** _____

3. Order: Unasyn (ampicillin) 50 mg/kg IV every 4 hours for infection

   Supply: Unasyn 1.5-g vial

   Nursing drug reference: Reconstitute each Unasyn 1.5-g vial with 4 mL
   of sterile water to yield 375 mg/mL.

   The child weighs 40 kg.

   ▶ **How many milliliters will you draw from the vial after
   reconstitution?** _____

4. Order: erythromycin 750 mg IV every 6 hours for infection

   Supply: erythromycin 1-g vial labeled: Reconstitute with 20 mL of sterile
   water for injection.

   ▶ **How many milliliters will you draw from the vial after
   reconstitution?** _____

5. Order: Fortaz 30 mg/kg IV every 8 hours for infection

   Supply: Fortaz 500-mg vial labeled: Reconstitute with 5 mL of sterile water
   for injection

   The child weighs 65 lb.

   ▶ **How many milliliters will you draw from the vial after
   reconstitution?** _____

■ MEDICATION PROBLEMS INVOLVING INTRAVENOUS PUMPS

IV medications are administered by drawing a specific amount of medication
from a vial or ampule and inserting that medication into an existing IV line. All
IV medications must be given with specific thought to exactly how much *time*
it should take to administer the medication. Information regarding time may be
obtained from a nursing drug reference, label, or package insert, or may be
specifically ordered by the physician.

Although IV medications can be administered IV push, the time involved
often requires the use of an IV pump. All IV pumps deliver milliliters per hour
(mL/hr) but may vary in operational capacity or size.

Below is an example of the dimensional analysis problem-solving method
with basic terms applied to a medication problem involving an IV pump.

Unit Path

Given Quantity	Conversion Factor for Given Quantity (Numerator)	Conversion Computation	Wanted Quantity
1500 Units	250 mL	15	
hr	25,000 Units	hr	= 15 mL

THINKING IT THROUGH

The two-factor–given quantity (the physician's order) contains a **numerator** (the dosage of medication) and a **denominator** (time). The wanted quantity (the answer to the problem) also contains a numerator (mL) and a denominator (time). This is called a two-factor–given quantity to a two-factor–wanted quantity medication problem. The denominator of the given quantity (hr) corresponds with the denominator of the wanted quantity (hr); therefore, only the numerator of the given quantity (units) needs to be canceled from the problem.

After factoring in the dose on hand, the unwanted unit (units) is canceled from the problem and the wanted unit (mL) remains in the numerator to correspond with the wanted quantity. The same number values are canceled from the numerator and denominator, leaving 15 mL/hr.

EXAMPLE 5.5

The physician orders heparin 1500 units/hr IV. The pharmacy sends an IV bag labeled: Heparin 25,000 units in 250 mL of D5W.

▶ Calculate the IV pump setting for milliliters per hour.

Given quantity   = 1500 units/hr
Wanted quantity = mL/hr
Dose on hand   = 25,000 units/250 mL

Sequential method:

STEP 1 Begin by identifying the given quantity. Establish the unit path to the wanted quantity.

Unit Path

Given Quantity	Conversion Factor for Given Quantity (Numerator)	Conversion Computation	Wanted Quantity
1500 Units / hr			= mL / hr

STEP 2

Unit Path

Given Quantity	Conversion Factor for Given Quantity (Numerator)	Conversion Computation	Wanted Quantity
1500 Units / hr	250 mL / 25,000 Units		= mL / hr

STEP 3

Unit Path

Given Quantity	Conversion Factor for Given Quantity (Numerator)	Conversion Computation	Wanted Quantity
1500 Units / hr	250 mL / 25,000 Units	15	= 15 mL / hr

▶▶▶ *15 mL/hr is the wanted quantity and the answer to the problem.*

EXAMPLE 5.6

The physician orders 500 mL of 0.45% NS with 20 mEq of KCl to infuse over 8 hours.

▶ **Calculate the number of milliliters per hour to set the IV pump.**

Given quantity   = 500 mL/8 hr
Wanted quantity = mL/hr

Sequential method:

$$\frac{500 \ \boxed{mL}}{8 \ \boxed{hr}} \bigg| \frac{500}{8} = \frac{62.5 \ mL}{} \ or \ \frac{63 \ mL}{hr}$$

▶▶▶ *63 mL/hr is the wanted quantity and the answer to the problem.*

EXAMPLE 5.7

The physician orders aminophylline 44 mg/hr IV. The pharmacy sends an IV bag labeled: Aminophylline 1 g/250 mL NS.

▶ **Calculate the milliliters per hour to set the IV pump.**

Given quantity   = 44 mg/hr
Wanted quantity = mL/hr
Dose on hand   = 1 g/250 mL

Random method:

$$\frac{44 \ \cancel{mg}}{\boxed{hr}} \bigg| \frac{250 \ \boxed{mL}}{\cancel{1 \ g}} \bigg| \frac{\cancel{1 \ g}}{1000 \ \cancel{mg}} \bigg| \frac{44 \times 25}{100} \bigg| \frac{1100}{100} = \frac{11 \ mL}{hr}$$

▶▶▶ *11 mL/hr is the wanted quantity and the answer to the problem.*

EXAMPLE 5.8

The nurse checks the IV pump and documents that the pump is set at and delivering 11 mL/hr and that the IV bag hanging is labeled: Aminophylline 1 g/250 mL.

▶ **How many milligrams per hour is the patient receiving?**

Given quantity   = 11 mL/hr
Wanted quantity = mg/hr
Dose on hand   = 1 g/250 mL

(Example continues on page 122)

Sequential method:

STEP 1

$$\frac{11 \text{ mL}}{\text{hr}} \huge| \normalsize = \frac{\text{mg}}{\text{hr}}$$

STEP 2

$$\frac{11 \text{ mL}}{\text{hr}} \Bigg| \frac{1 \text{ g}}{250 \text{ mL}} = \frac{\text{mg}}{\text{hr}}$$

STEP 3

$$\frac{11 \text{ mL}}{\text{hr}} \Bigg| \frac{1 \text{ g}}{250 \text{ mL}} \Bigg| \frac{1000 \text{ mg}}{1 \text{ g}} \Bigg| \frac{11 \times 100}{25} \Bigg| \frac{1100}{25} = \frac{44 \text{ mg}}{\text{hr}}$$

▶▶▶ *44 mg/hr is the wanted quantity and the answer to the problem.*

Exercise 5.3	**Medication Problems Involving Intravenous Pumps**

(See page 138 for answers)

1. Order: heparin 1800 units/hr IV

   Supply: heparin 25,000 units/250 mL D5W

   ▶ **Calculate the milliliters per hour to set the IV pump.** _____

2. Order: aminophylline 35 mg/hr IV

   Supply: aminophylline 1 g/250 mL NS

   ▶ **Calculate the milliliters per hour to set the IV pump.** _____

3. Information obtained by the nurse: heparin 25,000 units in 250 mL D5W is infusing at 30 mL/hr.

   ▶ **How many units per hour is the patient receiving?** _____

4. Information obtained by the nurse: aminophylline 1 g/250 mL NS is infusing at 15 mL/hr.

▶ **How many milligrams per hour is the patient receiving?** _____

5. Order: heparin 900 units/hr IV

Supply: heparin 25,000 units/500 mL D5W

▶ **Calculate the milliliters per hour to set the IV pump.** _____

■ MEDICATION PROBLEMS INVOLVING DROP FACTORS

Although IV pumps are used whenever possible, there are situations (no IV pumps available) and circumstances (outpatient or home care) that arise when IV pumps are not available and IV fluids or medications might be administered using gravity flow. **Gravity flow** involves calculating the drops per minute (gtt/min) required to infuse IV fluids or medications. When IV fluids or medications are administered using gravity flow, it is important to know the drop factor for the IV tubing that is being used. **Drop factor** is the drops per milliliter (gtt/mL) that the IV tubing will produce. Two types of IV tubing are available for gravity flow. *Macrotubing* delivers a large drop and is available in 10 gtt/mL, 15 gtt/mL, and 20 gtt/mL (Table 5.1); and *microtubing* delivers a small drop and is available in 60 gtt/mL.

Regardless of the IV tubing used, the problem can be solved by dimensional analysis. Below is an example of a medication problem involving drop factors using the dimensional analysis method.

PREVENTING MEDICATION ERRORS

When IV fluids are administered by gravity (without the use of an IV pump), it is the responsibility of the nurse to investigate the history of each patient to ensure safe delivery of IV fluids.

IV fluids that flow by gravity need to be monitored closely because the flow of the fluids can change with the position of the hand or arm. Some patients with a history of congestive heart failure do not tolerate large volumes of IV fluids.

Unit Path

Given Quantity	Conversion Factor for Given Quantity (Numerator)	Conversion Computation		Wanted Quantity
$\dfrac{250 \text{ mL}}{30 \text{ min}}$	$\dfrac{10 \text{ gtt}}{\text{mL}}$	$\dfrac{250 \times 1}{3}$	$\dfrac{250}{3} =$	$\dfrac{83.3 \text{ gtt}}{\text{min}}$ or $\dfrac{83 \text{ gtt}}{\text{min}}$

■ TABLE 5.1	Examples of Different Macrodrip Factors
MANUFACTURER	**DROPS PER MILLILITER (GTT/ML)**
Travenol	10
Abbott	15
McGaw	15
Cutter	20

THINKING IT THROUGH

The given quantity and the wanted quantity both include two factors; therefore, this is a two-factor–given quantity to a two-factor–wanted quantity medication problem.

The denominators are the same (min). The numerator in the given quantity (mL) is an unwanted unit and needs to be canceled.

When the drop factor is factored in, the unwanted unit (mL) is canceled, and the wanted unit (gtt) is placed in the numerator to correspond with the wanted quantity.

After you cancel the unwanted units from the problem, multiply the numerators, multiply the denominators, and divide the product of the numerators by the product of the denominators to provide the wanted quantity.

EXAMPLE 5.9

The physician orders 250 mL of normal saline to infuse in 30 minutes. The drop factor listed on the IV tubing box is 10 gtt/mL.

▶ **Calculate the number of drops per minute required to infuse the IV bolus.**

Given quantity   = 250 mL/30 min
Wanted quantity = gtt/min
Drop factor   = 10 gtt/mL

Sequential method:

STEP 1 Begin by identifying the given quantity and establishing a unit path to the wanted quantity.

Unit Path

Given Quantity	Conversion Factor for Given Quantity (Numerator)	Conversion Computation	Wanted Quantity
$\dfrac{250 \text{ mL}}{30 \text{ min}}$			$= \dfrac{\text{gtt}}{\text{min}}$

STEP 2

Unit Path

Given Quantity	Conversion Factor for Given Quantity (Numerator)	Conversion Computation	Wanted Quantity
$\dfrac{250 \text{ mL}}{30 \text{ min}}$	$\dfrac{10 \text{ gtt}}{\text{mL}}$		$= \dfrac{\text{gtt}}{\text{min}}$

STEP 3

Unit Path

Given Quantity	Conversion Factor for Given Quantity (Numerator)	Conversion Computation	Wanted Quantity
$\dfrac{250 \text{ mL}}{30 \text{ min}}$	$\dfrac{10 \text{ gtt}}{\text{mL}}$	$\dfrac{250 \times 1}{3} \quad \dfrac{250}{3}$	$= \dfrac{83.3 \text{ gtt}}{\text{min}} \text{ or } \dfrac{83 \text{ gtt}}{\text{min}}$

▶▶▶ *83 gtt is the wanted quantity and the answer to the problem.*

EXAMPLE 5.10

In some situations (home care), it may be important for the nurse to know exactly how long a specific amount of IV fluid will take to infuse. The physician may order a limited amount of IV fluid to infuse at a specific number of drops per minute (gtt/min).

The physician orders 1000 mL of D5W and 0.45% NS to infuse over 8 hours. The drop factor is 20 gtt/mL.

▶ **Calculate the number of drops per minute required to infuse the IV volume.**

Given quantity   = 1000 mL/8 hr
Wanted quantity = gtt/min
Drop factor   = 20 gtt/mL

Sequential method:

STEP 1

$$\frac{1000 \text{ mL}}{8 \text{ hr}} \cdot \frac{20 \text{ gtt}}{\text{mL}} = \frac{\text{gtt}}{\text{min}}$$

STEP 2

$$\frac{1000 \text{ mL}}{8 \text{ hr}} \cdot \frac{20 \text{ gtt}}{\text{mL}} \cdot \frac{1 \text{ hr}}{60 \text{ min}} = \frac{\text{gtt}}{\text{min}}$$

STEP 3

$$\frac{1000 \text{ mL}}{8 \text{ hr}} \cdot \frac{20 \text{ gtt}}{\text{mL}} \cdot \frac{1 \text{ hr}}{60 \text{ min}} \cdot \frac{1000 \times 2 \times 1}{8 \times 6} = \frac{2000}{48} = \frac{41.66 \text{ gtt}}{\text{min}}$$

$$\frac{41.66 \text{ gtt}}{\text{min}} \text{ or } \frac{42 \text{ gtt}}{\text{min}}$$

▶▶▶   *42 gtt/min is the wanted quantity and the answer to the problem.*

The unwanted unit (mL) is canceled, and the wanted unit (gtt) is placed in the numerator. Another unwanted unit (hr) needs to be canceled from the unit path.

The conversion factor (1 hr = 60 min) has been factored in to allow the unwanted unit (hr) to be canceled and the wanted unit (min) is placed in the denominator.

The given quantity and the wanted quantity have been identified and are both in the numerator; therefore, this is a one-factor–given quantity to a one-factor–wanted quantity medication problem.

The drop factor (10 gtt/mL) has been factored in using the sequential method to cancel the unwanted unit (mL).

The infusing rate of 21 gtt/min has now been factored in to cancel the unwanted unit (gtt).

The conversion factor (1 hr = 60 min) has been factored in to cancel the unwanted unit (min). The wanted unit (hr) remains in the numerator, which corresponds to the wanted quantity.

PREVENTING MEDICATION ERRORS

It is the responsibility of the nurse to ensure that an IV does not run dry and endanger the patient due to air in the IV line.

Check an IV bag infusing by gravity every 1 to 2 hours and/or instruct the patient to report when the IV has only a small amount (100 mL) left in the IV bag.

EXAMPLE 5.11

It is safe nursing practice to monitor an infusing IV every 2 hours to make sure it is infusing without difficulty and on time. It may be necessary to hang the next IV after $7\frac{1}{2}$ hours (before the estimated completion time) to keep the IV from running dry.

The physician orders 1000 mL of D5W. The drop factor is 10 gtt/mL. The infusion is dripping at 21 gtt/min.

▶ **How many hours will it take for the IV to infuse?**

Given quantity   = 1000 mL
Wanted quantity = hr
Drop factor   = 10 gtt/mL

STEP 1

$$\frac{1000 \text{ mL}}{} = \text{hr}$$

STEP 2

$$\frac{1000 \text{ mL}}{} \left| \frac{10 \text{ gtt}}{\text{mL}} \right. = \text{hr}$$

STEP 3

$$\frac{1000 \text{ mL}}{} \left| \frac{10 \text{ gtt}}{\text{mL}} \right| \frac{\text{min}}{21 \text{ gtt}} = \text{hr}$$

STEP 4

$$\frac{1000 \text{ mL}}{} \left| \frac{10 \text{ gtt}}{\text{mL}} \right| \frac{\text{min}}{21 \text{ gtt}} \left| \frac{1 \text{ hr}}{60 \text{ min}} \right. = \text{hr}$$

STEP 5

$$\frac{1000 \text{ mL}}{} \left| \frac{10 \text{ gtt}}{\text{mL}} \right| \frac{\text{min}}{21 \text{ gtt}} \left| \frac{1 \text{ hr}}{60 \text{ min}} \right| \frac{1000 \times 1 \times 1}{21 \times 6} \left| \frac{1000}{126} \right. = 7.93 \text{ hr or } 7.9 \text{ hr}$$

▶▶▶ *8 hours is the wanted quantity and the answer to the problem.*

Exercise 5.4   **Medication Problems Involving Drop Factors**
(See page 138 for answers)

1. Order: 800 mL D5W to infuse in 8 hours

   Drop factor: 15 gtt/mL

   ▶ **Calculate the number of drops per minute.** _____

2. Order: Infuse 250 mL NS

   Drop factor: 15 gtt/mL

   Infusion rate: 60 gtt/min

   ▶ **Calculate the hours to infuse.** _____

3. Order: 150 mL over 60 minutes

   Drop factor: 10 gtt/mL

   ▶ **Calculate the number of drops per minute.** _____

4. Order: 1000 mL D5W/0.9% NS

   Drop factor: 15 gtt/mL

   Infusion rate: 50 gtt/min

   ▶ **Calculate the number of hours to infuse.** _____

5. Order: 500 mL over 4 hours

   Drop factor: 15 gtt/mL

   ▶ **Calculate the number of drops per minute.** _____

PREVENTING MEDICATION ERRORS

When adding reconstituted medications to an IV solution, always check a nursing drug reference for compatibility of the solutions. To prevent precipitation and/or avoid extravasations, certain medications must be mixed in certain fluids and then further diluted.

Example: **Dilantin®** (phenytoin) must be reconstituted with normal saline (0.9% NaCl) and **never** administered into an IV line of dextrose in water (D₅W). Dilantin may only be further diluted with normal saline (0.9% NaCl).

Example: **Erythromycin** must be reconstituted with sterile water and may be further diluted in normal saline (0.9% NaCl) or dextrose in water (D₅W).

Example: **Acyclovir** must be reconstituted with sterile water and further diluted in varying strengths and combinations of normal saline (0.9% NaCl) and dextrose in water (D₅W).

■ MEDICATION PROBLEMS INVOLVING INTERMITTENT INFUSION

IV medications can be delivered over a specific amount of time by *intermittent infusion*. These medications require the use of an **infusion pump.** Some must be reconstituted and further diluted in a specific type and amount of IV fluid and delivered over a limited time. Others do not need to be reconstituted, but must be further diluted in a specific type and amount of IV fluid and delivered over a limited time.

EXAMPLE 5.12

The physician ordered erythromycin 500 mg IV every 6 hours for infection. The pharmacy sends a vial labeled: Erythromycin 1 g. The nursing drug reference provides information to reconstitute 1 g of erythromycin with 20 mL of sterile water and further dilute in 250 mL of 0.9% NS and to infuse over 1 hour.

▶ **How many milliliters will you draw from the vial after reconstitution?**

▶ **Calculate the milliliters per hour to set the IV pump.**

STEP 1

▶ **How many milliliters will you draw from the vial after reconstitution?**

Given quantity   = 500 mg
Wanted quantity = mL
Dose on hand   = 1 g/20 mL

Random method:

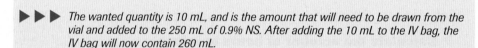

$$\frac{500 \text{ mg}}{} \left| \frac{20 \text{ mL}}{1 \text{ g}} \right| \frac{1 \text{ g}}{1000 \text{ mg}} \left| \frac{5 \times 2}{1} \right| \frac{10}{1} = 10 \text{ mL}$$

▶▶▶ *The wanted quantity is 10 mL, and is the amount that will need to be drawn from the vial and added to the 250 mL of 0.9% NS. After adding the 10 mL to the IV bag, the IV bag will now contain 260 mL.*

STEP 2

▶ **Calculate the milliliters per hour to set the IV pump.**

Given quantity   = 260 mL/1 hr
Wanted quantity = mL/hr

Sequential method:

$$\frac{260 \text{ mL}}{1 \text{ hr}} \left| \frac{260}{1} \right. = \frac{260 \text{ mL}}{\text{hr}}$$

▶▶▶ *The IV pump is set at 260 mL/hr to infuse the 500 mg of erythromycin ordered by the physician.*

STEP 2 (alternative): If an IV pump was unavailable, the infusion could be delivered by gravity using IV tubing with a drop factor of 10 gtt/mL.

▶ **Calculate the drops per minute required to infuse the IV volume.**

Given quantity   = 260 mL/1 hr
Wanted quantity = gtt/min
Drop factor   = 10 gtt/mL

Sequential method:

$$\frac{260 \text{ mL}}{1 \text{ hr}} \left| \frac{10 \text{ (gtt)}}{\text{mL}} \right| \frac{1 \text{ hr}}{60 \text{ (min)}} \left| \frac{260 \times 1 \times 1}{1 \times 6} \right| \frac{260}{6} = \frac{43.3 \text{ or } 43 \text{ gtt}}{\text{min}}$$

Exercise 5.5   **Medication Problems Involving Intermittent Infusion**
(See pages 138–139 for answers)

1. Order: ampicillin 250 mg IV every 4 hours for infection

   Supply: ampicillin 1-g vial

   Nursing drug reference: Reconstitute with 10 mL of 0.9% NS and further

   dilute in 50 mL NS. Infuse over 15 min.

   ▶ **How many milliliters will you draw from the vial after reconstitution?** _____

   ▶ **Calculate the milliliters per hour to set the IV pump.** _____

   ▶ **Calculate the drops per minute with a drop factor of 10 gtt/mL.** _____

2. Order: clindamycin 0.3 g IV every 6 hours for infection

   Supply: clindamycin 600 mg/4-mL vial

   Nursing drug reference: Dilute with 50 mL 0.9% NS and infuse over

   15 min.

   ▶ **How many milliliters will you draw from the vial?** _____

   ▶ **Calculate the milliliters per hour to set the IV pump.** _____

   ▶ **Calculate the drops per minute with a drop factor of 15 gtt/mL.** _____

(Exercise continues on page 130)

2. Order: meperidine 1.5 mg/kg PO every 4 hours for pain

   The child weighs 22 lb.

   ▶ **How many milliliters will you give?** _____

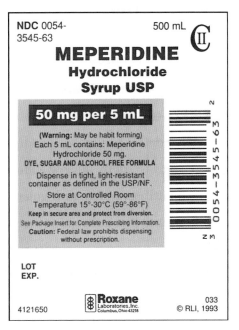

Courtesy of Roxane Laboratories.

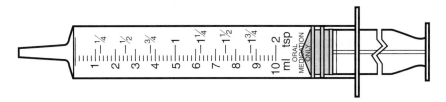

3. Order: Epogen 100 units/kg IV tid for anemia secondary to chronic renal

   failure

   The patient weighs 160 lb.

   ▶ **How many milliliters will you give?** _____

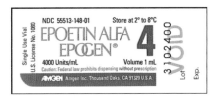

Courtesy of Amgen, Inc.

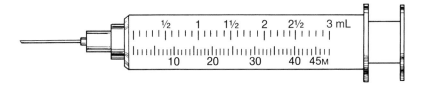

4. Order: Augmentin 10 mg/kg PO every 8 hours for otitis media

   Nursing drug reference: Dilute with 1 teaspoon (5 mL) of tap water

   and shake vigorously to yield 125 mg per 5 mL.

   The child weighs 25 kg.

   ▶ **How many milliliters will you give after**
     reconstitution? _____

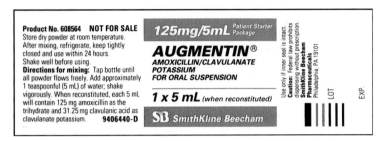

Courtesy of SmithKline Beecham Pharmaceuticals.

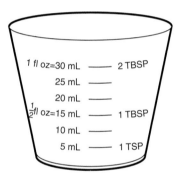

5. The physician orders heparin to infuse at 1300 units/hr continuous

   IV infusion.

   The pharmacy sends an IV bag labeled heparin 25,000 units in 250 mL.

   ▶ **Calculate the milliliters per hour to set the**
     IV pump. _____

6. A patient is receiving heparin 25,000 units in 250 mL infused at 25 mL/hr.

   ▶ **How many units per hour is the patient**
     receiving? _____

7. The physician orders morphine sulfate 2 mg/hr continuous IV for

   intractable pain related to end-stage lung cancer.

   The pharmacy sends an IV bag labeled morphine sulfate 100 mg in 250 mL.

   ▶ **Calculate the milliliters per hour to set the**
     IV pump. _____

8. Order: 1000 mL D5W/1/2 NS with 20 mEq of KCl to infuse in 12 hours

   Drop factor: 20 gtt/mL

   ▶ **Calculate the number of drops per minute.** _____

(Post-Test continues on page 136)

9. Order: Azactam 500 mg IV every 12 hours for septicemia

   Supply: Azactam 1-g vials

   Nursing drug reference: Dilute each 1-g vial with 10 mL of sterile water for injection and further dilute in 100 mL of NS to infuse over 60 minutes.

   ▶ **How many milliliters will you draw from the vial after reconstitution?** _____

   ▶ **Calculate the milliliters per hour to set the IV pump.** _____

   ▶ **Calculate the drops per minute with a drop factor of 20 gtt/mL.** _____

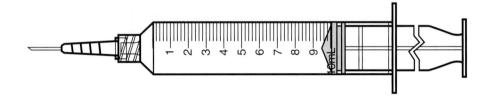

10. Order: Ancef 6.25 mg/kg IV every 6 hours for pneumonia

    The child weighs 38.2 kg.

    Nursing drug reference: Dilute each 1-g vial with 10 mL of sterile water for injection and further dilute 50 mL of NS to infuse over 30 minutes.

    ▶ **How many milliliters will you draw from the vial after reconstitution?** _____

    ▶ **Calculate the milliliters per hour to set the IV pump.** _____

    ▶ **Calculate the drops per minute with a drop factor of 10 gtt/mL.** _____

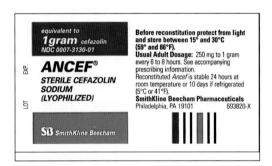

Courtesy of SmithKline Beecham Pharmaceuticals.

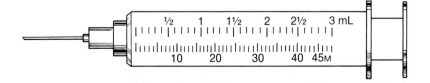

ANSWER KEY FOR CHAPTER 5: TWO-FACTOR MEDICATION PROBLEMS

Exercise 5.1 Pediatric Medication Problems Involving Weight

1. Sequential method:

$$\frac{1\ \text{mg}}{\text{kg}} \left| \frac{\text{mL}}{10\ \text{mg}} \right| \frac{1\ \text{kg}}{2.2\ \text{lb}} \left| \frac{45\ \text{lb}}{} \right| \frac{1 \times 1 \times 45}{10 \times 2.2} \left| \frac{45}{22} \right. = \begin{array}{l} 2.04\ \text{or} \\ 2\ \text{mL} \end{array}$$

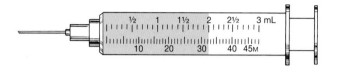

2. Sequential method:

$$\frac{0.01\ \text{mg}}{\text{kg}} \left| \frac{\text{mL}}{0.1\ \text{mg}} \right| \frac{1\ \text{kg}}{2.2\ \text{lb}} \left| \frac{20\ \text{lb}}{} \right| \frac{0.01 \times 1 \times 20}{0.1 \times 2.2} \left| \frac{0.2}{0.22} \right. = 0.9\ \text{mL}$$

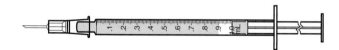

3. Sequential method:

$$\frac{0.5\ \text{mg}}{\text{kg}} \left| \frac{\text{mL}}{25\ \text{mg}} \right| \frac{1\ \text{kg}}{2.2\ \text{lb}} \left| \frac{45\ \text{lb}}{} \right| \frac{0.5 \times 1 \times 45}{25 \times 2.2} \left| \frac{22.5}{55} \right. = 0.4\ \text{mL}$$

4. Random method:

$$\frac{50\ \text{mcg}}{\text{kg}} \left| \frac{\text{mL}}{8\ \text{mg}} \right| \frac{1\ \text{mg}}{1000\ \text{mcg}} \left| \frac{1\ \text{kg}}{2.2\ \text{lb}} \right| \frac{75\ \text{lb}}{} \left| \frac{5 \times 1 \times 1 \times 75}{8 \times 100 \times 2.2} \right| \frac{375}{1760} = \text{mL}$$

$$\frac{375}{1760} = 0.2\ \text{mL}$$

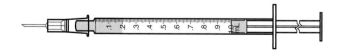

5. Random method:

$$\frac{10\ \text{mg}}{\text{kg}} \left| \frac{1\ \text{kg}}{2.2\ \text{lb}} \right| \frac{70\ \text{lb}}{} \left| \frac{5\ \text{mL}}{300\ \text{mg}} \right| \frac{10 \times 1 \times 7 \times 5}{2.2 \times 30} \left| \frac{350}{66} \right. = 5.3\ \text{or}\ 5\ \text{mL}$$

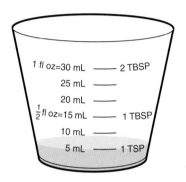

Exercise 5.2 Medication Problems Involving Reconstitution

1. Random method:

$$\frac{500\ \text{mg}}{} \left| \frac{50\ \text{mL}}{1\ \text{g}} \right| \frac{1\ \text{g}}{1000\ \text{mg}} \left| \frac{5 \times 5}{1} \right| \frac{25}{1} = 25\ \text{mL}$$

2. Sequential method:

$$\frac{250\ \text{mg}}{} \left| \frac{10\ \text{mL}}{500\ \text{mg}} \right| \frac{25 \times 1}{5} \left| \frac{25}{5} \right. = 5\ \text{mL}$$

3. Random method:

$$\frac{50\ \text{mg}}{\text{kg}} \left| \frac{4\ \text{mL}}{1.5\ \text{g}} \right| \frac{1\ \text{g}}{1000\ \text{mg}} \left| \frac{40\ \text{kg}}{} \right| \frac{5 \times 4 \times 1 \times 4}{1.5 \times 10} \left| \frac{80}{15} \right. = \begin{array}{l} 5.33\ \text{or} \\ 5\ \text{mL} \end{array}$$

Random method using yield:

$$\frac{50\ \text{mg}}{\text{kg}} \left| \frac{1\ \text{mL}}{375\ \text{mg}} \right| \frac{40\ \text{kg}}{} \left| \frac{50 \times 1 \times 40}{375} \right| \frac{2000}{375} = \begin{array}{l} 5.33\ \text{or} \\ 5\ \text{mL} \end{array}$$

4. Random method:

$$\frac{750\ \text{mg}}{} \left| \frac{20\ \text{mL}}{1\ \text{g}} \right| \frac{1\ \text{g}}{1000\ \text{mg}} \left| \frac{75 \times 2 \times 1}{1 \times 10} \right| \frac{150}{10} = 15\ \text{mL}$$

5. Sequential method:

$$\frac{30\text{ mg}}{\text{kg}}\left|\frac{5\ \text{(mL)}}{500\text{ mg}}\right|\frac{1\text{ kg}}{2.2\text{ lb}}\left|\frac{65\text{ lb}}{}\right|\frac{3\times5\times1\times65}{50\times2.2}\left|\frac{975}{110}\right|=\frac{8.86\text{ or}}{8.9\text{ mL}}$$

Exercise 5.3 Medication Problems Involving Intravenous Pumps

1. Sequential method:

$$\frac{1800\text{ units}}{\text{(hr)}}\left|\frac{250\ \text{(mL)}}{25,000\text{ units}}\right|\frac{18}{}=\frac{18\text{ mL}}{\text{hr}}$$

2. Random method:

$$\frac{35\text{ mg}}{\text{(hr)}}\left|\frac{250\ \text{(mL)}}{1\text{ g}}\right|\frac{1\text{ g}}{1000\text{ mg}}\left|\frac{35\times25}{100}\right|\frac{875}{100}=\frac{8.75\text{ or }9\text{ mL}}{\text{hr}}$$

3. Sequential method:

$$\frac{30\text{ mL}}{\text{(hr)}}\left|\frac{25,000\ \text{(units)}}{250\text{ mL}}\right|\frac{30\times2500}{25}\left|\frac{75,000}{25}\right|=\frac{3000\text{ units}}{\text{hr}}$$

4. Sequential method:

$$\frac{15\text{ mL}}{\text{(hr)}}\left|\frac{1\text{ g}}{250\text{ mL}}\right|\frac{1000\ \text{(mg)}}{1\text{ g}}\left|\frac{15\times100}{25}\right|\frac{1500}{25}=\frac{60\text{ mg}}{\text{hr}}$$

5. Sequential method:

$$\frac{900\text{ units}}{\text{(hr)}}\left|\frac{500\ \text{(mL)}}{25,000\text{ units}}\right|\frac{90\times5}{25}\left|\frac{450}{25}\right|=\frac{18\text{ mL}}{\text{hr}}$$

Exercise 5.4 Medication Problems Involving Drop Factors

1. Sequential method:

$$\frac{800\text{ mL}}{8\text{ hr}}\left|\frac{15\ \text{(gtt)}}{\text{mL}}\right|\frac{1\text{ hr}}{60\ \text{(min)}}\left|\frac{80\times15\times1}{8\times6}\right|\frac{1200}{48}=\frac{25\text{ gtt}}{\text{min}}$$

2. Sequential method:

$$\frac{250\text{ mL}}{}\left|\frac{15\text{ gtt}}{\text{mL}}\right|\frac{\text{min}}{60\text{ gtt}}\left|\frac{1\ \text{(hr)}}{60\text{ min}}\right|\frac{250\times15\times1}{60\times60}\left|\frac{3750}{3600}\right|=\frac{1.04\text{ or}}{1\text{ hr}}$$

3. Sequential method:

$$\frac{150\text{ mL}}{60\ \text{(min)}}\left|\frac{10\ \text{(gtt)}}{\text{mL}}\right|\frac{150\times1}{6}\left|\frac{150}{6}\right|=\frac{25}{\ }\frac{\text{gtt}}{\text{min}}$$

4. Sequential method:

$$\frac{1000\text{ mL}}{\text{mL}}\left|\frac{15\text{ gtt}}{50\text{ gtt}}\right|\frac{\text{min}}{60\text{ min}}\left|\frac{1\ \text{(hr)}}{5\times6}\right|\frac{10\times15\times1}{30}\left|\frac{150}{30}\right|=5\text{ hr}$$

5. Sequential method:

$$\frac{500\text{ mL}}{4\text{ hr}}\left|\frac{15\ \text{(gtt)}}{\text{mL}}\right|\frac{1\text{ hr}}{60\ \text{(min)}}\left|\frac{50\times15\times1}{4\times6}\right|\frac{750}{24}=\frac{31.25\text{ or }31}{\ }\frac{\text{gtt}}{\text{min}}$$

Exercise 5.5 Medication Problems Involving Intermittent Infusion

1. Random method:

$$\frac{250\text{ mg}}{}\left|\frac{10\ \text{(mL)}}{1\text{ g}}\right|\frac{1\text{ g}}{1000\text{ mg}}\left|\frac{25\times1}{10}\right|\frac{25}{10}=2.5\ \text{mL}$$

Calculate milliliters per hour to set the IV pump.
Sequential method:

$$\frac{50\ \text{(mL)}}{15\text{ min}}\left|\frac{60\text{ min}}{1\ \text{(hr)}}\right|\frac{50\times60}{15\times1}\left|\frac{3000}{15}\right|=\frac{200\text{ mL}}{\text{hr}}$$

Calculate drops per minute with a drop factor of 10 gtt/mL.
Sequential method:

$$\frac{50\text{ mL}}{15\ \text{(min)}}\left|\frac{10\ \text{(gtt)}}{\text{mL}}\right|\frac{50\times10}{15}\left|\frac{500}{15}\right|=\frac{33.33\text{ or }33}{\ }\frac{\text{gtt}}{\text{min}}$$

2. Random method:

$$\frac{0.3\text{ g}}{}\left|\frac{4\ \text{(mL)}}{600\text{ mg}}\right|\frac{1000\text{ mg}}{1\text{ g}}\left|\frac{0.3\times4\times10}{6\times1}\right|\frac{12}{6}=2\text{ mL}$$

Calculate milliliter per hour to set the IV pump.
Sequential method:

$$\frac{50\ \text{(mL)}}{15\text{ min}}\left|\frac{60\text{ min}}{1\ \text{(hr)}}\right|\frac{50\times60}{15\times1}\left|\frac{3000}{15}\right|=\frac{200\text{ mL}}{\text{hr}}$$

Calculate drops per minute with a drop factor of 15 gtt/mL.
Sequential method:

$$\frac{50 \text{ mL} \mid 15 \text{ gtt} \mid 50}{15 \text{ min} \mid \text{mL} \mid} = \frac{50}{} \frac{\text{gtt}}{\text{min}}$$

3. Sequential method:

$$\frac{3 \text{ g} \mid 40 \text{ mL} \mid 3 \times 40 \mid 120}{\mid 4 \text{ g} \mid 4 \mid 4} = 30 \text{ mL}$$

Calculate milliliters per hour to set the IV pump.
Sequential method:

$$\frac{130 \text{ mL} \mid 130}{1 \text{ hr} \mid 1} = \frac{130}{} \frac{\text{mL}}{\text{hr}}$$

Calculate drops per minute with a drop factor of 20 gtt/mL.
Sequential method:

$$\frac{130 \text{ mL} \mid 20 \text{ gtt} \mid 1 \text{ hr} \mid 130 \times 2 \mid 260}{1 \text{ hr} \mid \text{mL} \mid 60 \text{ min} \mid 6 \mid 6} = \frac{43.33 \text{ or } 43}{} \frac{\text{gtt}}{\text{min}}$$

4. Random method:

$$\frac{1000 \text{ mg} \mid 4 \text{ mL} \mid 1 \text{ g} \mid 4 \times 1 \mid 4}{\mid 1.5 \text{ g} \mid 1000 \text{ mg} \mid 1.5 \mid 1.5} = \frac{2.66 \text{ or}}{2.7 \text{ mL}}$$

Calculate milliliters per hour to set the IV pump.
Sequential method:

$$\frac{100 \text{ mL} \mid 100}{1 \text{ hr} \mid 1} = \frac{100}{} \frac{\text{mL}}{\text{hr}}$$

Calculate drops per minute with a drop factor of 20 gtt/mL.
Sequential method:

$$\frac{100 \text{ mL} \mid 20 \text{ gtt} \mid 1 \text{ hr} \mid 100 \times 2 \mid 200}{1 \text{ hr} \mid \text{mL} \mid 60 \text{ min} \mid 6 \mid 6} = \frac{33.33 \text{ or } 33}{} \frac{\text{gtt}}{\text{min}}$$

5. Sequential method:

$$\frac{50 \text{ mg} \mid \text{mL} \mid 50}{\mid 25 \text{ mg} \mid 25} = 2 \text{ mL}$$

Calculate milliliters per hour to set the IV pump.
Random method:

$$\frac{50 \text{ mL} \mid 60 \text{ min} \mid 50 \times 6 \mid 300}{30 \text{ min} \mid 1 \text{ hr} \mid 3 \times 1 \mid 3} = \frac{100}{} \frac{\text{mL}}{\text{hr}}$$

Calculate drops per minute with a drop factor of 10 gtt/mL.
Sequential method:

$$\frac{50 \text{ mL} \mid 10 \text{ gtt} \mid 50 \times 1 \mid 50}{30 \text{ min} \mid \text{mL} \mid 3 \mid 3} = \frac{16.66 \text{ or } 17}{} \frac{\text{gtt}}{\text{min}}$$

Practice Problems

1. Sequential method:

$$\frac{0.2 \text{ mg} \mid 2 \text{ mL} \mid 1 \text{ kg} \mid 10 \text{ lb} \mid 0.2 \times 2 \times 1 \times 10 \mid 4}{\text{kg} \mid 5 \text{ mg} \mid 2.2 \text{ lb} \mid \mid 5 \times 2.2 \mid 11} = \frac{0.36 \text{ or}}{0.4 \text{ mL}}$$

2. Sequential method:

$$\frac{10 \text{ mg} \mid 5 \text{ mL} \mid 8 \text{ kg} \mid 1 \times 5 \times 8 \mid 40}{\text{kg} \mid 160 \text{ mg} \mid \mid 16 \mid 16} = 2.5 \text{ mL}$$

3. Sequential method:

$$\frac{1.25 \text{ g} \mid 10 \text{ mL} \mid 1.25 \times 10 \mid 12.5}{\mid 2 \text{ g} \mid 2 \mid 2} = 6.25 \text{ or } 6.3 \text{ mL}$$

4. Random method:

$$\frac{750 \text{ mg} \mid 4 \text{ mL} \mid 1 \text{ g} \mid 75 \times 4 \times 1 \mid 300}{\mid 1.5 \text{ g} \mid 1000 \text{ mg} \mid 1.5 \times 100 \mid 150} = 2 \text{ mL}$$

5. Sequential method:

$$\frac{700 \text{ units} \mid 250 \text{ mL} \mid 7}{\text{hr} \mid 25,000 \text{ units} \mid} = \frac{7}{} \frac{\text{mL}}{\text{hr}}$$

or preparation by the nurse for immediate administration in a critical situation. The weight of the patient also may need to be obtained daily to ensure accurate correlation with the dosage of medication ordered. A nursing drug reference provides the nurse with information related to **dosage, weight,** and **time** for safe administration of medication.

To be able to calculate three-factor–given quantity to one-factor–, two-factor–, or three-factor–wanted quantity medication problems, it is necessary to understand all of the components of the medication order and to be able to calculate medication problems in a critical situation. This chapter will teach you to calculate medication problems involving the dosage of medication based on the weight of the patient and the time required for safe administration using dimensional analysis.

Three-factor–given quantity medication problems can be solved implementing the sequential method or the random method of dimensional analysis. The *given quantity* or the physician's order now contains three parts, including a **numerator** (the *dosage* of medication ordered) and two **denominators** (the *weight* of the patient and the *time* required for safe administration).

Below is an example of this problem-solving method showing placement of basic dimensional analysis terms applied to a three-factor medication problem.

Unit Path

Given Quantity	Conversion Factor for Given Quantity (Numerator)	Conversion Factor for Given Quantity (Denominator)	Conversion Computation	Wanted Quantity
30 mg	5 mL	22 kg	$30 \times 5 \times 22$	3300	11 mL
kg/day	300 mg		300	$\overline{300}$ =	day

EXAMPLE 6.1

The physician orders Tagamet for gastrointestinal ulcers 30 mg/kg/day PO in four divided doses for a child weighing 22 kg. The dose on hand is Tagamet 300 mg/5 mL.

▶ **How many milliliters per day will the child receive?**

Given quantity = 30 mg/kg/day
Wanted quantity = mL/day
Dose on hand   = 300 mg/5 mL
Weight   = 22 kg

STEP 1 Identify the three-factor–given quantity (the physician's order), which contains three parts: a *numerator* (30 mg) and two denominators (kg/day). Establish the unit path from the given *quantity* (30 mg/kg/day) to the *two-factor–wanted quantity* (mL/day) using the sequential method of dimensional analysis and the necessary conversion factors.

Sequential method:

$$\frac{30 \text{ mg}}{\text{kg/day}} \Bigg| \qquad\qquad\qquad\qquad\qquad = \frac{\text{mL}}{\text{day}}$$

STEP 2

Unit Path

Given Quantity	Conversion Factor for Given Quantity (Numerator)	Conversion Factor for Given Quantity (Denominator)	Conversion Computation	Wanted Quantity
30 ~~mg~~	5 (mL)			$= \dfrac{\text{mL}}{\text{day}}$
kg/(day)	300 ~~mg~~			

STEP 3

Unit Path

Given Quantity	Conversion Factor for Given Quantity (Numerator)	Conversion Factor for Given Quantity (Denominator)	Conversion Computation	Wanted Quantity
30 ~~mg~~	5 (mL)	22 ~~kg~~		$= \dfrac{\text{mL}}{\text{day}}$
~~kg~~/(day)	300 ~~mg~~			

STEP 4

Unit Path

Given Quantity	Conversion Factor for Given Quantity (Numerator)	Conversion Factor for Given Quantity (Denominator)	Conversion Computation		Wanted Quantity
~~30 mg~~	5 (mL)	22 ~~kg~~	$3 \times 5 \times 22$	330	11 mL
~~kg~~/(day)	300 ~~mg~~		30	30	$= \overline{\text{day}}$

(Example continues on page 144)

the wanted unit (mL) correlates with the *wanted quantity* (mL) and the unwanted unit (mg) is canceled.

The child's weight (22 kg) has been factored in and set up to allow the unwanted unit (kg) to be canceled.

All the unwanted units have been canceled, and the wanted units are placed to correlate with the two-factor–wanted quantity (mL/day). Multiply numerators, multiply denominators, and divide the product of the numerators by the product of the denominators to provide the numerical answer. The wanted quantity is 11 mL/day.

The child is to receive 11 mL/day in four divided doses; therefore, the *conversion factor* involves how many doses are in a day (4 divided doses = day).

STEP 5 **Using dimensional analysis, calculate how many milliliters per dose the child should receive.**

Given quantity   = 11 mL/day
Wanted quantity = mL/dose

$$\frac{11 \text{ mL}}{\text{day}} \;\Bigg| \hspace{3cm} = \frac{\text{mL}}{\text{dose}}$$

STEP 6

$$\frac{11\,\text{(mL)}}{\text{day}} \;\Bigg|\; \frac{\text{day}}{4\,\text{(doses)}} \;\Bigg|\; \frac{11}{4} = 2.75 \text{ or } \frac{2.8 \text{ mL}}{\text{dose}}$$

▶▶▶ *The wanted quantity is 2.8 mL/dose, and the child will receive this orally (PO) four times a day (qid).*

The problem could have been set up to find the wanted quantity of milliliters per dose.

STEP 6 (alternative).

Given quantity   = 30 mg/kg/day
Wanted quantity = mL/dose
Dose on hand   = 300 mg/5 mL
Weight   = 22 kg

Sequential method:

$$\frac{30\,\text{mg}}{\text{kg/day}} \;\Bigg|\; \frac{5\,\text{(mL)}}{300\,\text{mg}} \;\Bigg|\; \frac{22\,\text{kg}}{} \;\Bigg|\; \frac{\text{day}}{4\,\text{(doses)}} \;\Bigg|\; \frac{3 \times 5 \times 22}{30 \times 4} \;\Bigg|\; \frac{330}{120} = 2.75 \text{ or } \frac{2.8 \text{ mL}}{\text{dose}}$$

▶▶▶ *The wanted quantity is 2.8 mL/dose, and the child will receive this orally (PO) four times a day (qid).*

EXAMPLE 6.2

As a prudent nurse, you are concerned that the child may be receiving an unsafe dosage of Tagamet; therefore, you want to identify how many milligrams per kilogram per day (mg/kg/day) the child weighing 22 kg is receiving. The dosage of medication being given four times a day is 2.8 mL/dose. The dosage on hand is 300 mg/5 mL.

▶ **How many milligrams per kilogram per day is the child receiving?**

Given quantity   = 2.8 mL/dose
Wanted quantity = mg/kg/dose
Dose on hand   = 300 mg/5 mL
Child's weight   = 22 kg

PREVENTING MEDICATION ERRORS

Every new medication order for a child should be carefully reviewed for errors related to **dosage, route,** and **frequency.** Many **medication errors** can be eliminated if a double-check system is in place for all new medication orders.

THINKING IT THROUGH

The *two-factor–given quantity* (2.8 mL/dose) has been factored in with a *numerator* (2.8 mL) and a *denominator* (dose). The *three-factor–wanted quantity* (mg/kg/day) also has been factored in with a *numerator* (mg) and two *denominators* (kg/day).

The *conversion factors* have been added, and all

Sequential method:

STEP 1

$$\frac{2.8 \text{ mL}}{\text{dose}} \bigg| \qquad\qquad\qquad\qquad = \frac{\text{mg}}{\text{kg/day}}$$

STEP 2

$$\frac{2.8 \text{ mL}}{\text{dose}} \bigg| \frac{300 \text{ (mg)}}{5 \text{ mL}} \bigg| \frac{4 \text{ doses}}{\text{(day)}} \bigg| \frac{}{22 \text{ (kg)}} = \frac{\text{mg}}{\text{kg/day}}$$

STEP 3

$$\frac{2.8 \text{ mL}}{\text{dose}} \bigg| \frac{300 \text{ (mg)}}{5 \text{ mL}} \bigg| \frac{4 \text{ doses}}{\text{(day)}} \bigg| \frac{}{22 \text{ (kg)}} \bigg| \frac{2.8 \times 300 \times 4}{5 \times 22} \bigg| \frac{3360}{110} = \frac{30.54 \text{ or } 30.5 \text{ mg}}{\text{kg/day}}$$

▶▶▶ *The three-factor–wanted quantity is 30.5 mg/kg/day. The nursing drug reference identifies that 20 to 40 mg/kg/day in four divided doses is a safe dosage of Tagamet for children. Therefore, the nurse is assured that the child is receiving a correct dosage. Dimensional analysis assists you to critically think through any type of medication problem.*

EXAMPLE 6.3

The physician orders dobutamine 5 mcg/kg/min IV for cardiac failure. The pharmacy sends an IV bag labeled: dobutamine 250 mg/50 mL D5W/0.45% NS. The patient weighs 165 lb.

▶ **Calculate the milliliters per hour at which to set the IV pump.**

Given quantity = 5 mcg/kg/min
Wanted quantity = mL/hr
Dose on hand = 250 mg/50 mL
Weight = 165 lb

STEP 1 Identify the *three-factor–given quantity* (the physician's order) containing three parts, including the *numerator* (5 mg) and two *denominators* (kg/min). Establish the unit path from the three-factor–given quantity to the two-factor–wanted quantity (mL/hr).

Random method:

$$\frac{5 \text{ mcg}}{\text{kg/min}} \bigg| \qquad\qquad\qquad = \frac{\text{mL}}{\text{hr}}$$

(Example continues on page 146)

unwanted units have been canceled from the problem. The wanted unit (mg) is placed in the numerator to correlate with the *wanted quantity* (mg) also in the numerator. The wanted units (kg and day) are in the denominator to correlate with the wanted quantity (kg and day) in the denominator.

PREVENTING MEDICATION ERRORS

Knowing the **Six Rights** of medication administration can help to eliminate **medication errors** but another important consideration is being aware of the safe dosage range for each medication being administered.

A Nursing Drug Reference lists the safe dosage range for adults, children, and infants. It is the responsibility of the nurse to be familiar with safe dosage ranges to prevent **medication errors.**

THINKING IT THROUGH

The three-factor–given quantity has been set up with a *numerator* (5 mg) and *two denominators* (kg/min) leading across the unit path to a two-factor–wanted quantity with a *numerator* (mL) and a *denominator* (hr). By using the random method of

(Thinking it Through continues on page 146)

Dopamine Hydrochloride Injection, USP

DOSAGE AND ADMINISTRATION
WARNING: This is a potent drug. It must be diluted before administration to patient.
Suggested Dilution
Transfer contents of one or more additive syringes of dopamine hydrochloride by aseptic technique to either a 250 mL, or 500 mL container of one of the following sterile intravenous solutions:

1. Sodium Chloride Injection, USP
2. Dextrose 5% Injection, USP
3. Dextrose (5%) and Sodium Chloride (0.9%) Injection, USP
4. Dextrose (5%) and Sodium Chloride (0.45%) Injection, USP
5. Dextrose (5%) in Lactated Ringer's Injection
6. Sodium Lactate (1/6 Molar) Injection, USP
7. Lactated Ringer's Injection, USP

Dopamine HCl has been found to be stable for a minimum of 24 hours after dilution in the sterile intravenous solutions listed above. However, as with all intravenous admixtures, dilution should be made just prior to administration.

Do NOT add dopamine HCl to 5% Sodium Bicarbonate or other alkaline intravenous solution, since the drug is inactivated in alkaline solution.

Rate of Administration
Dopamine HCl, after dilution, is administered intravenously through a suitable intravenous catheter or needle. An IV drip chamber or other suitable metering device is essential for controlling the rate of flow in drops/minute. Each patient must be individually titrated to the desired hemodynamic and/or renal response with dopamine HCl. In titrating to the desired increase in systolic blood pressure, the optimum dosage rate for renal response may be exceeded, thus necessitating a reduction in rate after the hemodynamic condition is stabilized.

Administration at rates greater than 50 mcg/kg/minute have safely been used in advanced circulatory decompensation states. If unnecessary fluid expansion is of concern, adjustment of drug concentration may be preferred over increasing the flow rate of a less concentrated dilution.

Suggested Regimen
1. When appropriate, increase blood volume with whole blood or plasma until central venous pressure is 10 to 15 cm H_2O or pulmonary wedge pressure is 14 to 18 mm Hg.
2. Begin administration of diluted solution at doses of 2–5 mcg/kg/minute dopamine HCl in patients who are likely to respond to modest increments of heart force and renal perfusion.
   In more seriously ill patients, begin administration of diluted solution at doses of 5 mcg/kg/minute dopamine HCl and increase gradually using 5–10 mcg/kg/minute increments up to 20–50 mcg/kg/minute as needed. If doses of dopamine HCl in excess of 50 mcg/kg/minute are required, it is suggested that urine output be checked frequently. Should urine flow begin to decrease in the absence of hypotension, reduction of dopamine HCl dosage should be considered. Multiclinic trials have shown that more than 50% of the patients were satisfactorily maintained on doses of dopamine HCl of less than 20 mcg/kg/minute. In patients who do not respond to these doses with adequate arterial pressures or urine flow, additional increments of dopamine HCl may be employed in an effort to produce an appropriate arterial pressure and central perfusion.
3. Treatment of all patients requires constant evaluation of therapy in terms of the blood volume, augmentation of myocardial contractility, and distribution of peripheral perfusion. Dosage of dopamine HCl should be adjusted according to the patient's response, with particular attention to diminution of established urine flow rate, increasing tachycardia or development of new dysrhythmias as indices for decreasing or temporarily suspending the dosage.
4. As with all potent administered drugs, care should be taken to control the rate of administration to avoid inadvertent administration of a bolus of drug. Parenteral drug products should be inspected visually for particulate matter and discoloration prior to administration, whenever solution and container permit.

HOW SUPPLIED

Dopamine HCl 200 mg is supplied in the following form:	Dopamine HCl 800 mg is supplied in the following form:
Additive Syringe 5 mL (40 mg/mL) NDC 0186-0638-01	Additive Syringe 5 mL (160 mg/mL) NDC 0186-0642-01

Dopamine HCl 400 mg is supplied in the following forms:
Additive Syringe   5 mL (80 mg/mL)   NDC 0186-0641-01
                   10 mL (40 mg/mL)   NDC 0186-0639-01

Packages are color coded according to the total dosage content; 200 mg coded blue/white, 400 mg coded green/white and 800 mg coded yellow/white.

Store at controlled room temperature 15°–30°C (59°–86°F). Protect from light.

Avoid contact with alkalies (including sodium bicarbonate), oxidizing agents, or iron salts.

NOTE: Do not use the Injection if it is darker than slightly yellow or discolored in any way.

ASTRA® | Astra Pharmaceutical Products, Inc.
Westborough, MA 01581   021861R07   3/92 (7)

Courtesy of Astra Pharmaceutical Products.

7. Information obtained by the nurse: Nipride 50 mg/250 mL D5W is infusing at 22 mL/hr.

   Patient's weight: 160 lb

   ▶ **How many micrograms per kilogram per minute is the patient receiving?** _____

8. Order: Inocor 5 mcg/kg/min IV for congestive heart failure

   Supply: Inocor 100 mg/100 mL of 0.9% NS

   Patient's weight: 180 lb

   ▶ **Calculate the milliliters per hour to set the IV pump.** _____

9. Information obtained by the nurse: Nipride 50 mg/250 mL D5W is infusing at 46 mL/hr.

   Patient's weight: 160 lb

   ▶ **How many micrograms per kilogram per minute is the patient receiving?** _____

10. Order: bretylium 5 mg/kg in 50 mL D5W IV over 30 minutes for arrhythmia

    Supply: bretylium 500-mg vial

    Patient's weight: 240 lb

    ▶ **How many milliliters will you draw from the vial to equal 500 mg?** _____

    ▶ **Calculate the milliliters per hour to set the IV pump.** _____

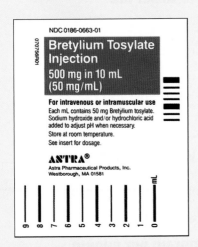

NDC 0186-0663-01

Bretylium Tosylate Injection
500 mg in 10 mL
(50 mg/mL)

For intravenous or intramuscular use
Each mL contains 50 mg Bretylium tosylate.
Sodium hydroxide and/or hydrochloric acid added to adjust pH when necessary.
Store at room temperature.
See insert for dosage.

ASTRA®
Astra Pharmaceutical Products, Inc.
Westborough, MA 01581

Courtesy of Astra Pharmaceutical Products.

Bretylium Tosylate Injection
For Intramuscular or Intravenous Use.

Suggested Bretylium Tosylate Admixture Dilutions and Administration Rates
for Continuous Infusion Maintenance Therapy Arranged in Descending Order of Concentration

PREPARATION				ADMINISTRATION		
Amount of Bretylium Tosylate	Volume of IV Fluid*	Final Volume	Final conc. (mg/mL)	Dose mg/min	Microdrops per min	mL/hour
FOR FLUID RESTRICTED PATIENTS:						
500 mg (10 mL)	50 mL	60 mL	8.3	1.0	7	7
				1.5	11	11
				2.0	14	14
2 g (40 mL)	500 mL	540 mL	3.7	1.0	16	16
1 g (20 mL)	250 mL	270 mL	3.7	1.5	24	24
				2.0	32	32
1 g (20 mL)	500 mL	520 mL	1.9	1.0	32	32
500 mg (10 mL)	250 mL	260 mL	1.9	1.5	47	47
				2.0	63	63

*IV fluid may be either Dextrose Injection, USP or Sodium Chloride Injection, USP. This table does not consider the overfill volume present in the IV fluids.

Courtesy of Astra Pharmaceutical Products.

Summary

This chapter has taught you to calculate three-factor medication problems involving the **dosage** of medication, the **weight** of the patient, and the amount of **time** over which medications or IV fluids can be safely administered. Using the sequential method or the random method of dimensional analysis, demonstrate your ability to calculate medication problems accurately by completing the following practice problems.

Practice Problems for Chapter 6	**Three-Factor Medication Problems** (See pages 164–165 for answers)

1. Order: amrinone 8 mcg/kg/min IV for congestive heart failure

   Supply: amrinone 100 mg/100 mL of 0.9% NS

   Patient's weight: 198 lb

   ▶ **Calculate the milliliters per hour to set the IV pump.** _____

2. Order: Tagamet 40 mg/kg/day PO in four divided doses for gastrointestinal ulcers

   Supply: Tagamet 300 mg/5 mL

   Child's weight: 80 lb

   ▶ **How many milliliters per dose will you give?** _____

3. Information obtained by the nurse: dopamine 200 mg in 500 mL D5W is infusing at 45 mL/hr for a patient weighing 60 kg.

   ▶ **How many micrograms per kilogram per minute is the patient receiving?** _____

4. Order: dopamine 2 mcg/kg/min IV for decreased cardiac output

   Supply: dopamine 400 mg/500 mL

   Patient's weight: 176 lb

   ▶ **Calculate the milliliters per hour to set the IV pump.** _____

5. Order: Neupogen 5 mcg/kg/day SQ for 2 weeks for neutropenia

   Supply: Neupogen 300 mcg/mL

   Patient's weight: 130 lb

   ▶ **How many micrograms per day will you give?** _____

6. Order: aminophylline 0.5 mg/kg/hr IV loading dose for bronchodilation

   Supply: aminophylline 250 mg/250 mL D5W

   Patient's weight: 132 lb

   ▶ **Calculate the milliliters per hour to set the IV pump. _____**

7. Order: furosemide 2 mg/kg/day PO for congestive heart failure

   Supply: furosemide 10 mg/mL

   Child's weight: 40 kg

   ▶ **How many milliliters per day will you give? _____**

8. Information obtained by the nurse: Nipride 200 mg in 1000 mL D5W is

   infusing at 15 mL/hr for a patient weighing 100 kg.

   ▶ **How many micrograms per kilogram per minute is the patient receiving? _____**

9. Information obtained by the nurse: A child weighing 65 lb is receiving

   10 mL of Tagamet PO qid from a stock bottle labeled: Tagamet

   300 mg/5 mL.

   ▶ **How many milligrams per kilogram per day is the child receiving? _____**

10. Information obtained by the nurse: aminophylline 250 mg/250 mL 0.9%

    NS is infusing at 25 mL/hr for a patient weighing 50 kg.

    ▶ **How many milligrams per kilogram per hour is the patient receiving? _____**

Chapter 6 Post-Test:
Three-Factor Medication Problems

Name _____   **Date** _____

1. Order: morphine sulfate 0.3 mg/kg/dose PO every 4 hours for pain

   Supply: morphine sulfate 10 mg/5 mL

   Child's weight: 20 lb

   ▶ **How many milliliters per dose will you give?** _____

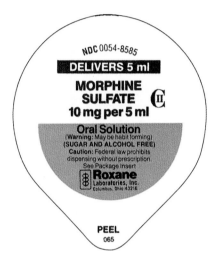

NDC 0054-8585

DELIVERS 5 ml

MORPHINE SULFATE C-II
10 mg per 5 ml

Oral Solution
(Warning: May be habit forming)
(SUGAR AND ALCOHOL FREE)
Caution: Federal law prohibits
dispensing without prescription.
See Package Insert
Roxane
Laboratories, Inc.
Columbus, Ohio 43216

PEEL
065

Courtesy of Roxane Laboratories, Inc.

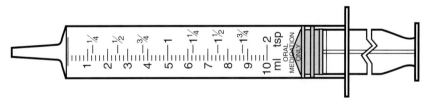

(Post-Test continues on page 158)

2. Order: filgrastim 5 mcg/kg/day for myelosuppression secondary to chemotherapy administration

Supply: filgrastim 480 mcg/1.6 mL

Patient's weight: 100 lb

▶ **How many milliliters per day will you give?** _____

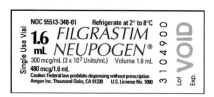

Courtesy of Amgen, Inc.

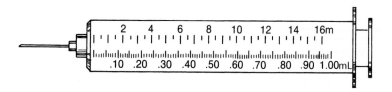

3. Order: Epogen 100 units/kg/day SQ three times weekly for anemia secondary to AZT administration

Supply: Epogen 10,000 units/mL

Patient's weight: 180 lb

▶ **How many milliliters per day will you give?** _____

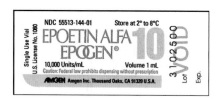

Courtesy of Amgen, Inc.

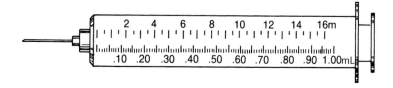

4. Order: digoxin 25 mcg/kg/day PO every 8 hours for congestive heart
   failure

   Supply: digoxin 0.25 mg/5 mL

   Child's weight: 25 lb

▶ **How many milliliters will you give per day?** _____

▶ **How many milliliters will you give per dose?** _____

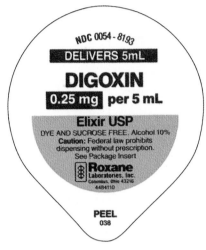

Courtesy of Roxane Laboratories, Inc.

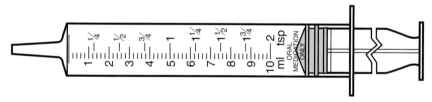

(Post-Test continues on page 160)

5. Order: clindamycin 10 mg/kg/day IV in three divided doses for
respiratory tract infection

Supply: clindamycin 150 mg/mL

Child's weight: 10 kg

▶ **How many milliliters per dose will you draw from
the vial?** _____

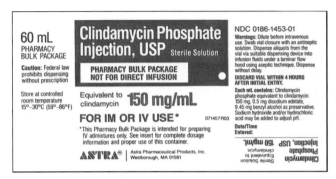

Courtesy of Astra Pharmaceutical Products.

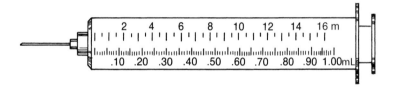

6. Order: Claforan 100 mg/kg/day IV in two divided doses for infection

Supply: Claforan 1 g/10 mL

Neonate's weight: 2045 g

▶ **How many milliliters per dose will you draw from
the vial?** _____

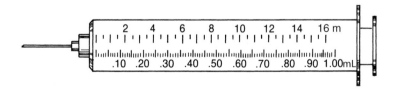

7. Order: gentamicin 2.5 mg/kg/dose IV every 12 hours for gram-negative
bacillary infection

Supply: gentamicin 40 mg/mL

Neonate's weight: 1182 g

▶ **How many milligrams per dose will the
neonate receive?** _____

8. Order: ampicillin 100 mg/kg/day IV in divided doses every 12 hours for respiratory tract infection

Supply: ampicillin 125 mg/5 mL

Neonate's weight: 1182 g

▶ **How many milligrams per dose will the neonate receive?** _____

▶ **How many milliliters per dose will you draw from the vial?** _____

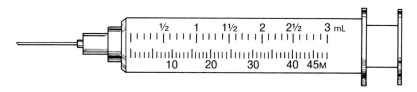

9. Order: Solu-Medrol 5.4 mg/kg/hr IV for acute spinal cord injury

Supply: Solu-Medrol 125 mg/2 mL

Patient's weight: 160 lb

▶ **How many milligrams per hour will the patient receive?** _____

10. Order: aminophylline 0.8 mg/kg/hr IV for respiratory distress

Supply: aminophylline 250 mg/100 mL

Child's weight: 65 lb

▶ **Calculate the milliliters per hour to set the IV pump.** _____

ANSWER KEY FOR CHAPTER 6: THREE-FACTOR MEDICATION PROBLEMS

Exercise 6.1 Medication Problems Involving Dosage, Weight, and Time

1. Sequential method:

$$\frac{2 \text{ mg}}{\text{kg/day}}\left|\frac{5 \text{ (mL)}}{40 \text{ mg}}\right|\frac{20 \text{ kg}}{}\left|\frac{\text{day}}{2 \text{ (doses)}}\right|\frac{2 \times 5 \times 2}{4 \times 2}\left|\frac{20}{8}\right| = \frac{2.5 \text{ mL}}{\text{dose}}$$

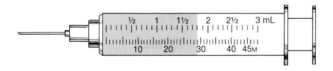

2. Random method:

$$\frac{40 \text{ mg}}{\text{kg/day}}\left|\frac{10 \text{ (mL)}}{1 \text{ g}}\right|\frac{\text{day}}{3 \text{ (doses)}}\left|\frac{1 \text{ kg}}{2.2 \text{ lb}}\right|\frac{30 \text{ lb}}{}\left|\frac{1 \text{ g}}{1000 \text{ mg}}\right| = \frac{\text{mL}}{\text{dose}}$$

$$\frac{4 \times 1 \times 3}{3 \times 2.2}\left|\frac{12}{6.6}\right| = \frac{1.81 \text{ or } 1.8 \text{ mL}}{\text{dose}}$$

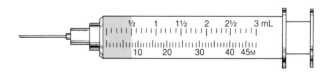

3. Sequential method:

$$\frac{6 \text{ mg}}{\text{kg/day}}\left|\frac{5 \text{ (mL)}}{125 \text{ mg}}\right|\frac{1 \text{ kg}}{2.2 \text{ lb}}\left|\frac{45 \text{ lb}}{}\right|\frac{\text{day}}{2 \text{ (doses)}} = \frac{\text{mL}}{\text{dose}}$$

$$\frac{6 \times 5 \times 1 \times 45}{125 \times 2.2 \times 2}\left|\frac{1350}{550}\right| = \frac{2.45 \text{ or } 2.5 \text{ mL}}{\text{dose}}$$

4. Sequential method:

$$\frac{1.5 \text{ mg}}{\text{kg/day}}\left|\frac{5 \text{ (mL)}}{6.7 \text{ mg}}\right|\frac{20 \text{ kg}}{}\left|\frac{\text{day}}{4 \text{ (doses)}}\right|\frac{1.5 \times 5 \times 20}{6.7 \times 4} = \frac{\text{mL}}{\text{dose}}$$

$$\frac{150}{26.8} = \frac{5.59 \text{ or } 5.6 \text{ mL}}{\text{dose}}$$

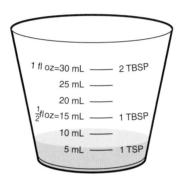

5. Sequential method:

$$\frac{10 \text{ mg}}{\text{kg/day}}\left|\frac{2 \text{ (mL)}}{300 \text{ mg}}\right|\frac{1 \text{ kg}}{2.2 \text{ lb}}\left|\frac{1 \text{ day}}{3 \text{ (doses)}}\right|\frac{50 \text{ lb}}{}\left|\frac{1 \times 2 \times 1 \times 1 \times 5}{3 \times 2.2 \times 3}\right|\frac{10}{19.8} = \frac{0.5 \text{ mL}}{\text{dose}}$$

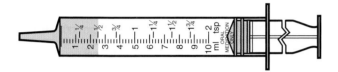

6. Sequential method:

$$\frac{400 \text{ mg}}{}\left|\frac{\text{(mL)}}{40 \text{ mg}}\right|\frac{40}{4} = 10 \text{ mL}$$

Random method:

$$\frac{5 \text{ mcg}}{\text{kg/min}}\left|\frac{60 \text{ min}}{1 \text{ (hr)}}\right|\frac{1 \text{ kg}}{2.2 \text{ lb}}\left|\frac{200 \text{ lb}}{}\right|\frac{260 \text{ (mL)}}{400 \text{ mg}}\left|\frac{1 \text{ mg}}{1000 \text{ mcg}}\right| = \frac{\text{mL}}{\text{hr}}$$

$$\frac{5 \times 6 \times 2 \times 26 \times 1}{2.2 \times 4 \times 10}\left|\frac{1560}{88}\right| = \frac{17.7 \text{ or } 18 \text{ mL}}{\text{hr}}$$

Practice Problems

Practice Problems **One–Factor Practice Problems**
(See pages 203–206 for answers)

1. Order: Tigan 200 mg qid IM for nausea and vomiting

▶ **How many milliliters will you give?** _____

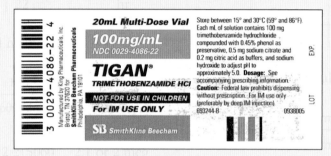

Courtesy of SmithKline Beecham Pharmaceuticals.

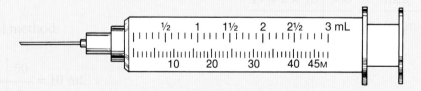

2. Order: morphine 30 mg PO every 4 hours for pain

▶ **How many tablets will you give?** _____

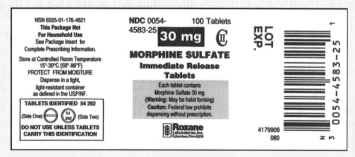

Courtesy of Roxane Laboratories.

3. Order: prednisone 7.5 mg PO bid for inflammation

▶ **How many tablets will you give?** _____

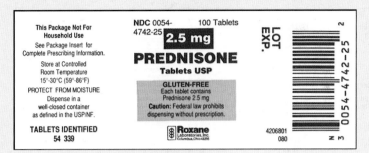

Courtesy of Roxane Laboratories.

4. Order: acetaminophen 160 mg PO every 4 hours for fever

▶ **How many teaspoons will you give?** _____

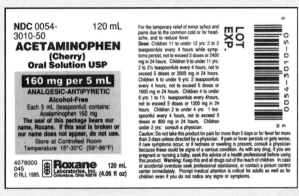

Courtesy of Roxane Laboratories.

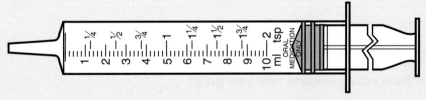

(Practice Problems continue on page 168)

5. Order: Xanax 0.5 mg PO tid for anxiety

▶ **How many tablets will you give?** _____

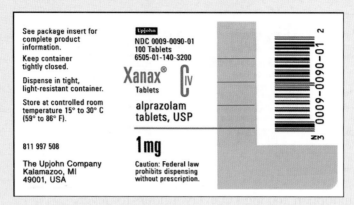

Courtesy of the Upjohn Company.

6. Order: Adalat 60 mg PO daily for hypertension

▶ **How many tablets will you give?** _____

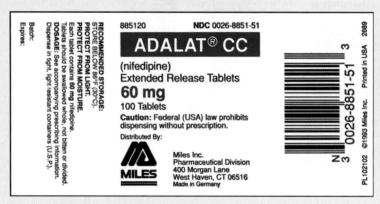

Courtesy of Miles Inc.

7. Order: Halcion 0.25 mg PO at hs for insomnia

▶ **How many tablets will you give?** _____

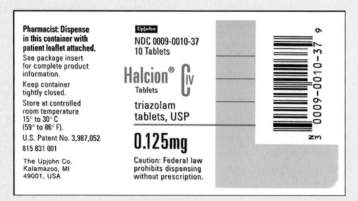

Courtesy of the Upjohn Company.

8. Order: furosemide 80 mg PO daily for congestive heart failure

▶**How many tablets will you give?** _____

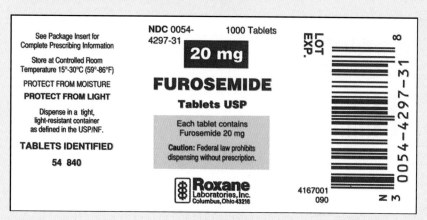

See Package Insert for
Complete Prescribing Information

Store at Controlled Room
Temperature 15°-30°C (59°-86°F)

PROTECT FROM MOISTURE

PROTECT FROM LIGHT

Dispense in a tight,
light-resistant container
as defined in the USP/NF.

TABLETS IDENTIFIED

54 840

NDC 0054-4297-31   1000 Tablets

20 mg

FUROSEMIDE

Tablets USP

Each tablet contains
Furosemide 20 mg

Caution: Federal law prohibits
dispensing without prescription.

✚ **Roxane**
Laboratories, Inc.
Columbus, Ohio 43216

4167001
090

Courtesy of Roxane Laboratories.

9. Order: morphine sulfate 10 mg IM prn for pain

▶**How many milliliters will you give?** _____

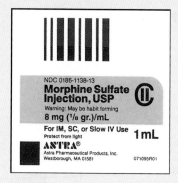

NDC 0186-1138-13
**Morphine Sulfate
Injection, USP** Ⓒ
Warning: May be habit forming
8 mg (¹/₈ gr.)/mL
For IM, SC, or Slow IV Use **1 mL**
Protect from light
ASTRA®
Astra Pharmaceutical Products, Inc.
Westborough, MA 01581   071095R01

Courtesy of Astra Pharmaceutical Products.

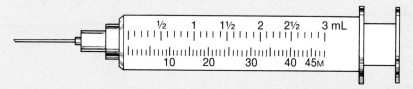

(Practice Problems continue on page 170)

10. Order: naloxone HCl 100 mcg IVP prn for respiratory depression

▶ **How many milliliters will you give?** _____

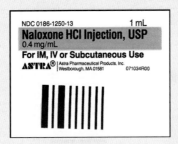

NDC 0186-1250-13   1 mL
Naloxone HCl Injection, USP
0.4 mg/mL
For IM, IV or Subcutaneous Use
ASTRA® | Astra Pharmaceutical Products, Inc.
            | Westborough, MA 01581   071034R00

Courtesy of Astra Pharmaceutical Products.

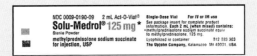

11. Order: Solu-Medrol 80 mg IVP every 4 hours for inflammation

▶ **How many milliliters will you give?** _____

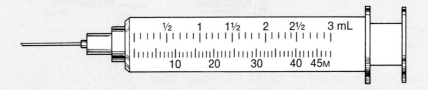

NDC 0009-0190-09   2 mL Act-O-Vial®   Single-Dose Vial   For IV or IM use
Solu-Medrol® 125 mg *
Sterile Powder
methylprednisolone sodium succinate
for injection, USP
The Upjohn Company, Kalamazoo MI 49001, USA

Courtesy of the Upjohn Company.

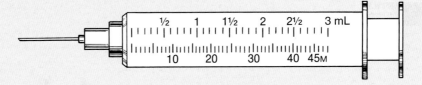

12. Order: lactulose 20 g PO daily for constipation

▶ **How many milliliters will you give?** _____

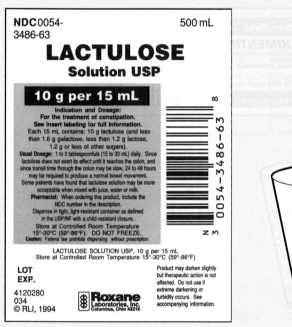

Courtesy of Roxane Laboratories.

13. Order: Compazine 5 mg IM tid for nausea and vomiting

▶ **How many milliliters will you give?** _____

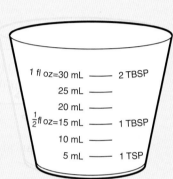

Courtesy of SmithKline Beecham Pharmaceuticals.

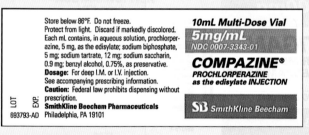

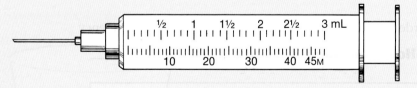

(Practice Problems continue on page 172)

19. Order: magnesium sulfate 1000 mg IM times four doses for hypomagnesemia

▶ **How many milliliters will you give?** _____

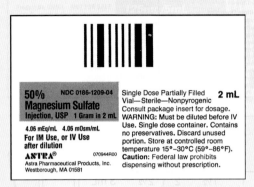

> **50%**
> **Magnesium Sulfate**
> Injection, USP   1 Gram in 2 mL
>
> NDC 0186-1209-04
>
> 4.06 mEq/mL   4.06 mOsm/mL
> **For IM Use, or IV Use**
> **after dilution**
> **ASTRA®**   070944R00
> Astra Pharmaceutical Products, Inc.
> Westborough, MA 01581
>
> Single Dose Partially Filled   **2 mL**
> Vial—Sterile—Nonpyrogenic
> Consult package insert for dosage.
> WARNING: Must be diluted before IV
> Use. Single dose container. Contains
> no preservatives. Discard unused
> portion. Store at controlled room
> temperature 15°–30°C (59°–86°F).
> **Caution:** Federal law prohibits
> dispensing without prescription.

Courtesy of Astra Pharmaceutical Products.

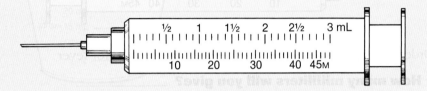

20. Order: Compazine 10 mg PO qid prn for nausea and vomiting

▶ **How many teaspoons will you give?** _____

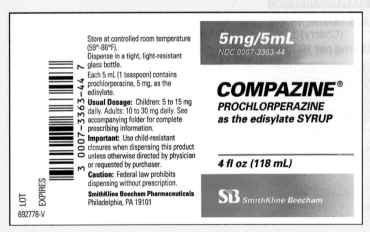

> Store at controlled room temperature
> (59°-86°F).
> Dispense in a tight, light-resistant
> glass bottle.
> Each 5 mL (1 teaspoon) contains
> prochlorperazine, 5 mg, as the
> edisylate.
> **Usual Dosage:** Children: 5 to 15 mg
> daily. Adults: 10 to 30 mg daily. See
> accompanying folder for complete
> prescribing information.
> **Important:** Use child-resistant
> closures when dispensing this product
> unless otherwise directed by physician
> or requested by purchaser.
> **Caution:** Federal law prohibits
> dispensing without prescription.
> **SmithKline Beecham Pharmaceuticals**
> Philadelphia, PA 19101
>
> LOT
> EXPIRES
> 692778-V
>
> 3 0007-3363-44 7
>
> **5mg/5mL**
> NDC 0007-3363-44
>
> **COMPAZINE®**
> PROCHLORPERAZINE
> as the edisylate SYRUP
>
> **4 fl oz (118 mL)**
>
> **SB** SmithKline Beecham

Courtesy of SmithKline Beecham Pharmaceuticals.

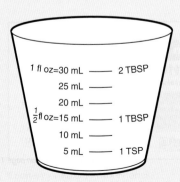

> 1 fl oz=30 mL ——— 2 TBSP
> 25 mL ———
> 20 mL ———
> ½ fl oz=15 mL ——— 1 TBSP
> 10 mL ———
> 5 mL ——— 1 TSP

21. Order: Hemabate 0.25 mg IM to control postpartum bleeding

▶ **How many milliliters will you give?** _____

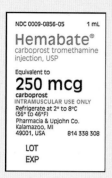

NDC 0009-0856-05   1 mL

Hemabate®
carboprost tromethamine
injection, USP

Equivalent to
250 mcg
carboprost
INTRAMUSCULAR USE ONLY
Refrigerate at 2° to 8°C
(36° to 46°F)
Pharmacia & Upjohn Co.
Kalamazoo, MI
49001, USA   814 338 308

LOT
EXP

Courtesy of Pharmacia & Upjohn Company.

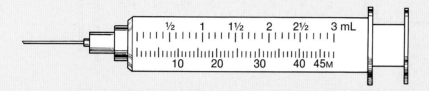

22. Order: Lincocin 500 mg every 8 hours IV for infection

▶ **How many milliliters will you draw
from the vial?** _____

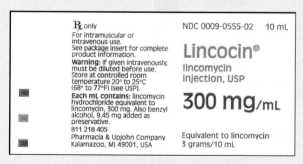

℞ only
For intramuscular or
intravenous use.
See package insert for complete
product information.
Warning: If given intravenously,
must be diluted before use.
Store at controlled room
temperature 20° to 25°C
(68° to 77°F) [see USP].
Each mL contains: lincomycin
hydrochloride equivalent to
lincomycin, 300 mg. Also benzyl
alcohol, 9.45 mg added as
preservative.
811 218 405
Pharmacia & Upjohn Company
Kalamazoo, MI 49001, USA

NDC 0009-0555-02   10 mL

Lincocin®
lincomycin
injection, USP

300 mg/mL

Equivalent to lincomycin
3 grams/10 mL

Courtesy of Pharmacia & Upjohn Company.

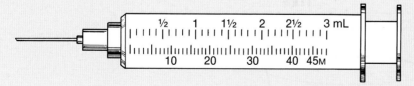

(Practice Problems continue on page 176)

23. Order: Fragmin 2500 IU SQ daily for 10 days for thromboembolism
prophylaxis

▶ **How many milliliters will you give?** _____

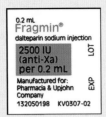

Courtesy of Pharmacia & Upjohn Company.

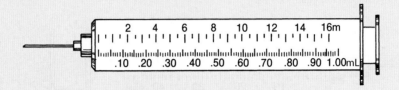

24. Order: Vantin 200 mg every 12 hours PO for infection

▶ **How many milliliters will you give?** _____

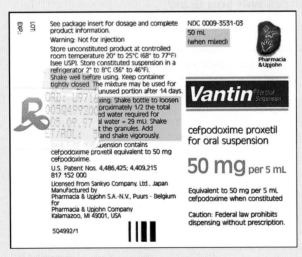

Courtesy of Pharmacia & Upjohn Company.

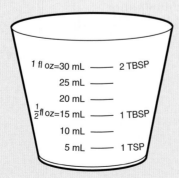

25. Order: Cleocin 300 mg PO daily for *P. carinii* pneumonia

▶ **How many capsules will you give?** _____

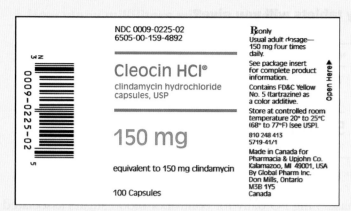

Courtesy of Pharmacia & Upjohn Company.

26. Order: Azulfidine 500 mg PO every 12 hours for management of

inflammatory bowel disease

▶ **How many tablets will you give?** _____

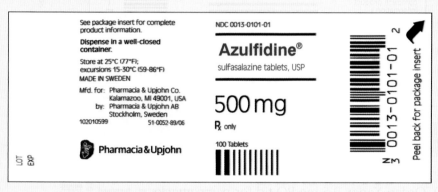

Courtesy of Pharmacia & Upjohn Company.

27. Order: Mirapex 0.25 mg PO tid for signs/symptoms of idiopathic

Parkinson's disease

▶ **How many tablets will you give?** _____

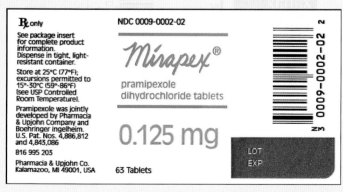

Courtesy of Pharmacia & Upjohn Company.

(Practice Problems continue on page 178)

33. Order: Phenobarbital 60 mg PO bid for seizures

    Supply: Phenobarbital Elixir 20 mg/5 mL

    ▶ **How many milliliters will you give?** _____

34. Order: Abacavir (Ziagen) 600 mg PO every day for HIV-1 infection in

    combination with Zidovudine

    Supply: Ziagen 300 mg/tablets

    ▶ **How many tablets will you give?** _____

35. Order: Zidovudine 100 mg PO every four hours for symptomatic HIV

    infection (600 mg/daily total)

    Supply: Zidovudine 10 mg/mL syrup

    ▶ **How many milliliters will you give?** _____

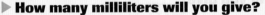

Practice Problems	**Two-Factor Practice Problems**

(See pages 206–209 for answers)

1. Order: digoxin elixir 25 mcg/kg for congestive heart failure

    Child's weight: 25 lb

    ▶ **How many milliliters will you give?** _____

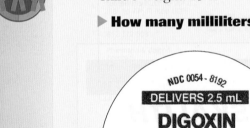

NDC 0054 - 8192

DELIVERS 2.5 mL

DIGOXIN

0.125 mg per 2.5 mL

Elixir USP

DYE AND SUCROSE FREE, Alcohol 10%
Caution: Federal law prohibits
dispensing without prescription.
See Package Insert

Roxane
Laboratories, Inc.
Columbus, Ohio 43216
4484100

PEEL
038

Courtesy of Roxane Laboratories.

2. Order: atropine sulfate 0.02 mg/kg IV every 4 hours for bradycardia

Child's weight: 35 lb

▶ **How many milliliters will you give?** _____

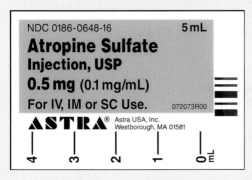

NDC 0186-0648-16   5 mL

Atropine Sulfate
Injection, USP

0.5 mg (0.1 mg/mL)

For IV, IM or SC Use.   072073R00

ASTRA® Astra USA, Inc.
Westborough, MA 01581

4   3   2   1   0 mL

Courtesy of Astra Pharmaceutical Products.

3. Order: lidocaine 2 mg/min IV for arrhythmia

Supply: lidocaine 2 g/500 mL D5W

▶ **Calculate the milliliters per hour to set
the IV pump.** _____

4. Order: Mezlin 1.5 g IV every 4 hours for infection

Nursing drug reference: Reconstitute each 1 g with 10 mL of normal saline.

▶ **How many milliliters will you draw from the vial
alter reconstitution?** _____

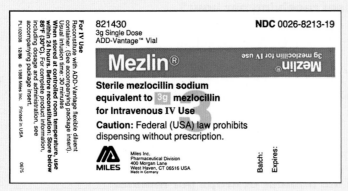

For IV Use
Reconstitute with ADD-Vantage flexible diluent
container (See accompanying package insert).
Usual infusion time 30 minutes
When stored at controlled room temperature, use
within 24 hours. Before reconstitution: Store below
86°F (30°C). For complete product information,
including dosage and administration, see
accompanying package insert.

PL102038 12/88 © 1988 Miles Inc. Printed in USA 0675

821430
3g Single Dose
ADD-Vantage™ Vial

NDC 0026-8213-19

Mezlin®

Sterile mezlocillin sodium
equivalent to 3g mezlocillin
for Intravenous IV Use

Caution: Federal (USA) law prohibits
dispensing without prescription.

MILES   Miles Inc.
Pharmaceutical Division
400 Morgan Lane
West Haven, CT 06516 USA
Made in Germany

Batch:

Expires:

Courtesy of Miles.

5. Order: gentamicin 1 mg/kg IV every 8 hours for infection

Supply: gentamicin 40 mg/mL

Child's weight: 94 lb

▶ **How many milliliters will you draw
from the vial?** _____

(Practice Problems continue on page 182)

6. Order: morphine 15 mg/hr IV for intractable pain

Supply: morphine 300 mg/500 mL NS

▶ **Calculate the milliliters per hour to set the IV pump.** _____

7. Information obtained by the nurse: Dilaudid 50 mg in 250 mL NS is infusing at 25 mL/hr.

▶ **How many milligrams per hour is the patient receiving?** _____

8. Order: add 10 mEq KCl to 1000 mL D5W

Supply: KCl 20 mEq/20 mL

▶ **How many milliliters will you draw from the vial to add to the IV bag?** _____

9. Information obtained by the nurse: nitroglycerin 50 mg in 500 mL D5W is infusing at 3 mL/hr.

▶ **How many micrograms per minute is the patient receiving?** _____

10. Information obtained by the nurse: 1000 mL D5W with 10 mEq KCl is infusing at 100 mL/hr.

▶ **How many milliequivalents of KCl is the patient receiving per hour?** _____

11. Order: infuse 1000 mL D5W at 250 mL/hr

Drop factor: 20 gtt/mL

▶ **Calculate the number of drops per minute.** _____

12. Order: infuse 750 mL NS over 5 hours

Drop factor: 10 gtt/mL

▶ **Calculate the number of drops per minute.** _____

13. Order: infuse 500 mL D5W over 8 hours

Drop factor: 60 gtt/mL

▶ **Calculate the number of drops per minute.** _____

14. Order: infuse 750 mL D5W

Drop factor: 15 gtt/mL

Infusion rate: 18 gtt/min

▶ **Calculate the number of hours to infuse.** _____

15. Order: infuse 250 mL NS

    Drop factor: 15 gtt/mL

    Infusion rate: 50 gtt/min

    ▶ **Calculate the number of hours to infuse.** _____

16. Order: infuse 1000 mL D5W/0.45% NS

    Drop factor: 15 gtt/mL

    Infusion rate: 25 gtt/min

    ▶ **Calculate the number of hours to infuse.** _____

17. Order: Fortaz 1.25 g IV every 12 hours for urinary tract infection

    Supply: Fortaz 2-g vial

    Nursing drug reference: Dilute each 1 g with 10 mL of sterile water and

    further dilute in 100 mL 0.9% NS to infuse over 1 hour.

    ▶ **How many milliliters will you draw from the vial
    after reconstitution?** _____

    ▶ **Calculate the milliliters per hour
    to set the IV pump.** _____

    ▶ **Calculate the drops per minute with a drop factor
    of 10 gtt/mL.** _____

18. Order: vancomycin 275 mg IV every 8 hours for infection

    Supply: vancomycin 500-mg vial

    Nursing drug reference: Reconstitute each 500-mg vial with 10 mL NS

    and further dilute with 250 mL NS to infuse over 1 hour.

    ▶ **How many milliliters will you draw from the vial
    after reconstitution?** _____

    ▶ **Calculate the milliliters per hour to set the
    IV pump.** _____

    ▶ **Calculate the drops per minute with a drop factor
    of 10 gtt/mL.** _____

(Practice Problems continue on page 184)

19. Order: Mezlin 450 mg IV every 4 hours for infection

    Supply: Mezlin 4-g vial

    Nursing drug reference: Reconstitute each 1 g with 10 mL of sterile water and further dilute in 100 mL NS to infuse over 30 minutes.

    ▶ **How many milliliters will you draw from the vial after reconstitution?** _____

    ▶ **Calculate the milliliters per hour to set the IV pump.** _____

    ▶ **Calculate the drops per minute with a drop factor of 10 gtt/mL.** _____

20. Order: gentamicin 23 mg IV every 8 hours for infection

    Supply: gentamicin 40 mg/mL

    Nursing drug reference: Dilute with 100 mL NS and infuse over 1 hour.

    ▶ **How many milliliters will you draw from the vial after reconstitution?** _____

    ▶ **Calculate the milliliters per hour to set the IV pump.** _____

    ▶ **Calculate the drops per minute with a drop factor of 15 gtt/mL.** _____

21. Order: Cortef 0.56 mg/kg PO daily for adrenal insufficiency

    ▶ **How many milliliters will you give a child weighing 18 kg?** _____

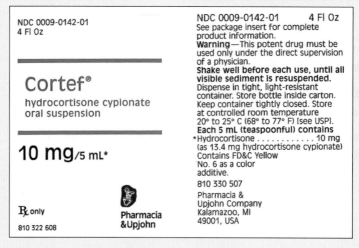

NDC 0009-0142-01
4 Fl Oz

Cortef®
hydrocortisone cypionate
oral suspension

10 mg/5 mL*

℞ only
810 322 608

**Pharmacia
&Upjohn**

NDC 0009-0142-01   4 Fl Oz
See package insert for complete product information.
Warning—This potent drug must be used only under the direct supervision of a physician.
Shake well before each use, until all visible sediment is resuspended.
Dispense in tight, light-resistant container. Store bottle inside carton. Keep container tightly closed. Store at controlled room temperature 20° to 25° C (68° to 77° F) [see USP].
Each 5 mL (teaspoonful) contains
*Hydrocortisone . . . . 10 mg (as 13.4 mg hydrocortisone cypionate)
Contains FD&C Yellow No. 6 as a color additive.
810 330 507
Pharmacia & Upjohn Company
Kalamazoo, MI 49001, USA

Courtesy of Pharmacia & Upjohn Company.

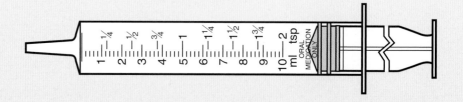

22. Order: Colestid 30 g/day PO in four divided doses for hyper-

cholesterolemia or management of cholesterol

▶ **How many packets/dose will you give?** _____

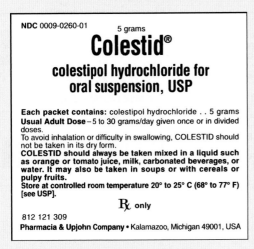

NDC 0009-0260-01   5 grams

Colestid®

colestipol hydrochloride for oral suspension, USP

Each packet contains: colestipol hydrochloride . . 5 grams
Usual Adult Dose – 5 to 30 grams/day given once or in divided doses.
To avoid inhalation or difficulty in swallowing, COLESTID should not be taken in its dry form.
COLESTID should always be taken mixed in a liquid such as orange or tomato juice, milk, carbonated beverages, or water. It may also be taken in soups or with cereals or pulpy fruits.
Store at controlled room temperature 20° to 25° C (68° to 77° F) [see USP].

℞ only

812 121 309
Pharmacia & Upjohn Company • Kalamazoo, Michigan 49001, USA

Courtesy of Pharmacia & Upjohn Company.

23. Order: vincristine 10 mcg/kg IV weekly for treatment of Hodgkin's

lymphoma

▶ **How many milliliters will you give a patient weighing 50 kg?** _____

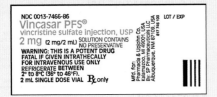

NDC 0013-7466-86   LOT / EXP
Vincasar PFS®
vincristine sulfate injection, USP
2 mg (2 mg/2 mL) SOLUTION CONTAINS NO PRESERVATIVE
WARNING: THIS IS A POTENT DRUG FATAL IF GIVEN INTRATHECALLY FOR INTRAVENOUS USE ONLY
REFRIGERATE BETWEEN 2° to 8°C (36° to 46°F).
2 mL SINGLE DOSE VIAL ℞ only
Mfd. for: Pharmacia & Upjohn Co. Kalamazoo, MI 49001, USA By: SP Pharmaceuticals LLC Albuquerque, NM 87109, USA

Courtesy of Pharmacia & Upjohn Company.

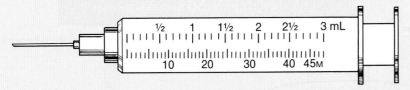

(Practice Problems continue on page 186)

24. Order: Tagamet 1600 mg/day PO in two divided doses for gastro-esophageal reflux disease

▶ **How many tablets per dose will you give?** _____

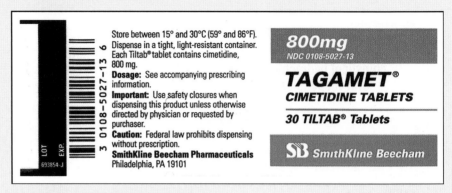

Store between 15° and 30°C (59° and 86°F). Dispense in a tight, light-resistant container. Each Tiltab® tablet contains cimetidine, 800 mg.
Dosage: See accompanying prescribing information.
Important: Use safety closures when dispensing this product unless otherwise directed by physician or requested by purchaser.
Caution: Federal law prohibits dispensing without prescription.
SmithKline Beecham Pharmaceuticals
Philadelphia, PA 19101

800mg
NDC 0108-5027-13

TAGAMET®
CIMETIDINE TABLETS

30 TILTAB® Tablets

SB SmithKline Beecham

Courtesy of SmithKline Beecham Pharmaceuticals.

25. Order: Thorazine 1 g/day PO in three divided doses for psychoses

▶ **How many milliliters per dose will you give?** _____

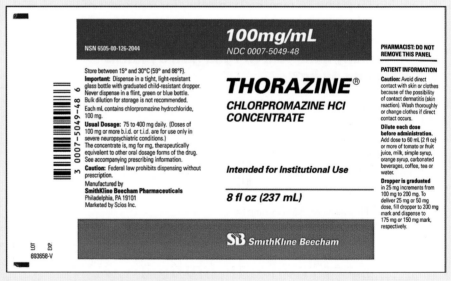

NSN 6505-00-126-2044

100mg/mL
NDC 0007-5049-48

Store between 15° and 30°C (59° and 86°F).
Important: Dispense in a tight, light-resistant glass bottle with graduated child-resistant dropper. Never dispense in a flint, green or blue bottle. Bulk dilution for storage is not recommended.
Each mL contains chlorpromazine hydrochloride, 100 mg.
Usual Dosage: 75 to 400 mg daily. (Doses of 100 mg or more b.i.d. or t.i.d. are for use only in severe neuropsychiatric conditions.)
The concentrate is, mg for mg, therapeutically equivalent to other oral dosage forms of the drug. See accompanying prescribing information.
Caution: Federal law prohibits dispensing without prescription.
Manufactured by
SmithKline Beecham Pharmaceuticals
Philadelphia, PA 19101
Marketed by Scios Inc.

THORAZINE®
CHLORPROMAZINE HCl
CONCENTRATE

Intended for Institutional Use

8 fl oz (237 mL)

SB SmithKline Beecham

PHARMACIST: DO NOT REMOVE THIS PANEL

PATIENT INFORMATION
Caution: Avoid direct contact with skin or clothes because of the possibility of contact dermatitis (skin reaction). Wash thoroughly or change clothes if direct contact occurs.

Dilute each dose before administration. Add dose to 60 mL (2 fl oz) or more of tomato or fruit juice, milk, simple syrup, orange syrup, carbonated beverages, coffee, tea or water.

Dropper is graduated in 25 mg increments from 100 mg to 200 mg. To deliver 25 mg or 50 mg dose, fill dropper to 200 mg mark and dispense to 175 mg or 150 mg mark, respectively.

Courtesy of SmithKline Beecham Pharmaceuticals.

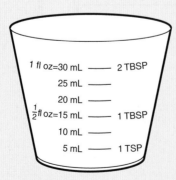

1 fl oz=30 mL —— 2 TBSP
25 mL ——
20 mL ——
½ fl oz=15 mL —— 1 TBSP
10 mL ——
5 mL —— 1 TSP

26. Order: Epivir 4 mg/kg PO bid for treatment of HIV infection

▶ **How many milliliters will you give a child weighing 20 kg?** _____

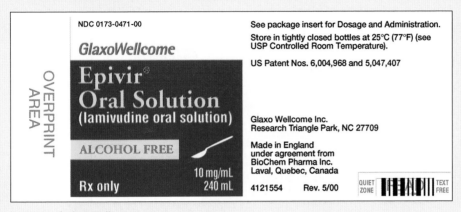

NDC 0173-0471-00

GlaxoWellcome

Epivir®
Oral Solution
(lamivudine oral solution)

ALCOHOL FREE

Rx only   10 mg/mL
              240 mL

OVERPRINT AREA

See package insert for Dosage and Administration.
Store in tightly closed bottles at 25°C (77°F) (see USP Controlled Room Temperature).

US Patent Nos. 6,004,968 and 5,047,407

Glaxo Wellcome Inc.
Research Triangle Park, NC 27709

Made in England
under agreement from
BioChem Pharma Inc.
Laval, Quebec, Canada

4121554   Rev. 5/00

Courtesy of GlaxoWellcome.

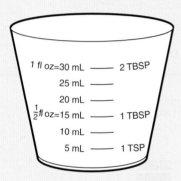

1 fl oz=30 mL ——— 2 TBSP
25 mL ———
20 mL ———
½ fl oz=15 mL ——— 1 TBSP
10 mL ———
5 mL ——— 1 TSP

27. Order: Zofran 0.15 mg/kg IV 15 to 30 minutes before administration

of chemotherapy for prevention of nausea and vomiting

▶ **How many milliliters will you give a patient weighing 160 lb?** _____

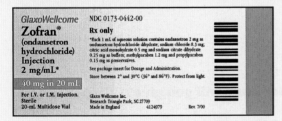

GlaxoWellcome
Zofran®
(ondansetron
hydrochloride)
Injection
2 mg/mL*

40 mg in 20 mL

For I.V. or I.M. Injection.
Sterile
20-mL Multidose Vial

NDC 0173-0442-00

Rx only

*Each 1 mL of aqueous solution contains ondansetron 2 mg as ondansetron hydrochloride dihydrate; sodium chloride 8.3 mg; citric acid monohydrate 0.5 mg and sodium citrate dihydrate 0.25 mg as buffers; methylparaben 1.2 mg and propylparaben 0.15 mg as preservatives.

See package insert for Dosage and Administration.

Store between 2° and 30°C (36° and 86°F). Protect from light.

Glaxo Wellcome Inc.
Research Triangle Park, NC 27709
Made in England   4124979   Rev. 7/00

Courtesy of GlaxoWellcome.

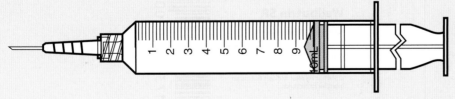

(Practice Problems continue on page 188)

28. Order: Epivir 2 mg/kg PO twice daily for treatment of HIV infection

▶ **How many tablets will you give a patient weighing 40 kg?** _____

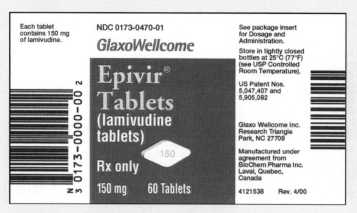

Courtesy of GlaxoWellcome.

29. Order: Zovirax 20 mg/kg PO qid for 5 days for treatment of chickenpox

▶ **How many tablets will you give a child weighing 20 lb?** _____

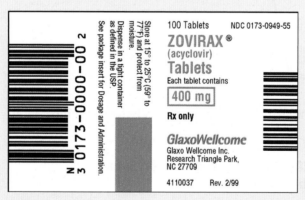

Courtesy of GlaxoWellcome.

30. Order: Wellbutrin SR 450 mg/day PO in three divided doses for treatment of depression

▶ **How many tablets per dose will you give?** _____

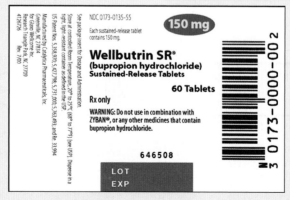

Courtesy of GlaxoWellcome.

31. Order: Zantac 2.4 g/day PO in four divided doses for treatment of duodenal ulcer

▶ **How many tablets per dose will you give?** _____

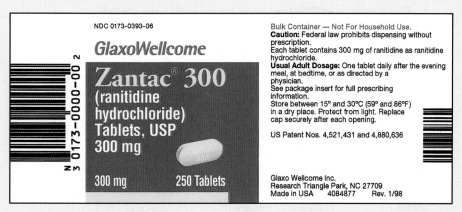

NDC 0173-0393-06

GlaxoWellcome

Zantac® 300
(ranitidine
hydrochloride)
Tablets, USP
300 mg

300 mg   250 Tablets

N 3 0173-0000-00 2

Bulk Container — Not For Household Use.
Caution: Federal law prohibits dispensing without prescription.
Each tablet contains 300 mg of ranitidine as ranitidine hydrochloride.
Usual Adult Dosage: One tablet daily after the evening meal, at bedtime, or as directed by a physician.
See package insert for full prescribing information.
Store between 15° and 30°C (59° and 86°F) in a dry place. Protect from light. Replace cap securely after each opening.

US Patent Nos. 4,521,431 and 4,880,636

Glaxo Wellcome Inc.
Research Triangle Park, NC 27709
Made in USA   4084877   Rev. 1/98

Courtesy of GlaxoWellcome.

32. Order: Zinacef 500 mg/day IV in two divided doses for urinary tract infection

▶ **How many milliliters per dose will you give?** _____

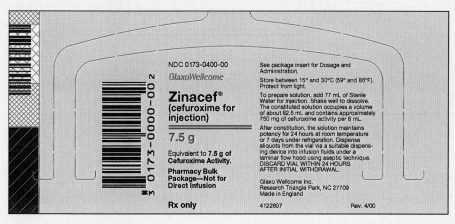

NDC 0173-0400-00

GlaxoWellcome

Zinacef®
(cefuroxime for
injection)

7.5 g

Equivalent to 7.5 g of
Cefuroxime Activity.

Pharmacy Bulk
Package—Not for
Direct Infusion

Rx only

N 2 0173-0000-00 2

See package insert for Dosage and Administration.
Store between 15° and 30°C (59° and 86°F). Protect from light.

To prepare solution, add 77 mL of Sterile Water for Injection. Shake well to dissolve. The constituted solution occupies a volume of about 82.5 mL and contains approximately 750 mg of cefuroxime activity per 8 mL.

After constitution, the solution maintains potency for 24 hours at room temperature or 7 days under refrigeration. Dispense aliquots from the vial via a suitable dispensing device into infusion fluids under a laminar flow hood using aseptic technique. DISCARD VIAL WITHIN 24 HOURS AFTER INITIAL WITHDRAWAL.

Glaxo Wellcome Inc.
Research Triangle Park, NC 27709
Made in England

4122607   Rev. 4/00

Courtesy of GlaxoWellcome.

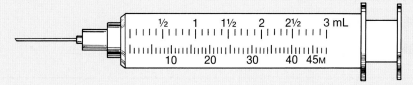

(Practice Problems continue on page 190)

33. Order: Ceptaz 1000 mg/day IV in two divided doses for treatment of respiratory tract infection

    Nursing drug reference: Dilute each 1-g vial with 10 mL of normal saline.

    ▶ **How many milliliters per dose will you give?** _____

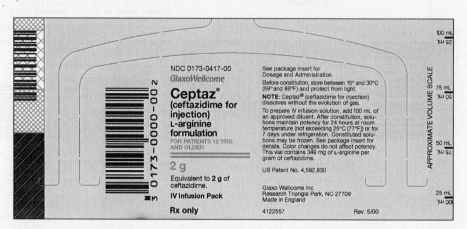

Courtesy of GlaxoWellcome.

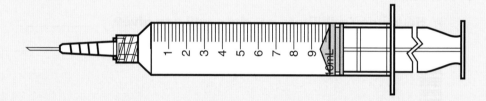

34. Order: Gantrisin 150 mg/2.2 lb PO divided into 5 doses given over 24 hours for urinary tract infection

    Child's weight: 30 kg

    ▶ **How many milliliters per dose will you give?** _____

35. Order: Abacavir (Ziagen) 8 mg/kg PO bid for HIV-1 infection in combination with Zidovudine

    Supply: Ziagen 20 mg/mL oral solution

    Child's weight: 40 kg

    ▶ **How many milliliters will you give?** _____

Practice Problems **Three-Factor Practice Problems**
(See pages 209–212 for answers)

1. Order: Tagamet 40 mg/kg/day PO in four divided doses for treatment of active ulcer

Child's weight: 60 kg

▶ **How many milliliters per day will you give?** _2400_

▶ **How many milliliters per dose will you give?** _200_

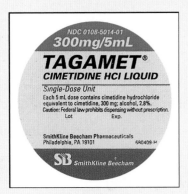

Courtesy of SmithKline Beecham Pharmaceuticals.

2. Order: furosemide 4 mg/kg/day IV for management of hypercalcemia of malignancy

Child's weight: 60 lb

▶ **How many milliliters per day will you give?** _____

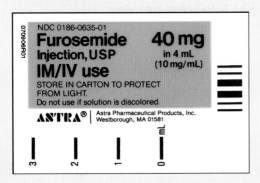

Courtesy of Astra Pharmaceutical Products.

(Practice Problems continue on page 192)

3. Order: Cleocin 30 mg/kg/day IV in divided doses every 8 hours

for infection

Child's weight: 50 kg

▶ **How many milliliters per day will you give?** _____

▶ **How many milliliters per dose will you give?** _____

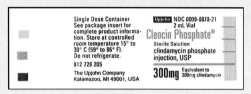

Single Dose Container
See package insert for
complete product informa-
tion. Store at controlled
room temperature 15° to
30° C (59° to 86° F).
Do not refrigerate.

812 728 205

The Upjohn Company
Kalamazoo, MI 49001, USA

Upjohn NDC 0009-0870-21
2 mL Vial
Cleocin Phosphate®
Sterile Solution
clindamycin phosphate
injection, USP

300mg   Equivalent to
300mg clindamycin

Courtesy of the Upjohn Company.

4. Information obtained by the nurse: A child is receiving 0.575 mL/dose

of gentamicin IV every 8 hours from a supply of gentamicin 40 mg/mL.

Child's weight: 45 lb

▶ **How many milligrams per kilogram per day
is the patient receiving?** _____

5. Information obtained by the nurse: A child is receiving 0.125 mL/dose

of diphenhydramine (Benadryl) IV every 8 hours from a supply of

Benadryl 50 mg/mL.

Child's weight: 20 lb

▶ **How many milligrams per kilogram per day
is the child receiving?** _____

6. Order: dopamine 5 mcg/kg/min IV for decreased cardiac output

   Supply: dopamine 400-mg vial

   Nursing drug reference: Dilute each 400-mg vial in 250 mL NS

   Patient's weight: 110 lb

   ▶ **How many milliliters will you draw from the vial?** _____

   ▶ **Calculate the milliliters per hour to set the IV pump.** _____

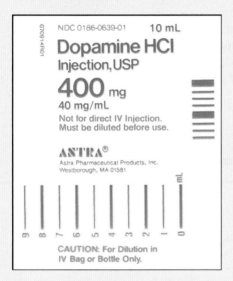

Courtesy of Astra Pharmaceutical Products.

7. Order: Nipride 0.8 mcg/kg/min IV for hypertensive crisis

   Supply: Nipride 50 mg/500 mL NS

   Patient's weight: 143 lb

   ▶ **Calculate the milliliters per hour to set the IV pump.** _____

8. Information obtained by the nurse: Nipride 50 mg in 250 mL NS is

   infusing at 68 mL/hr.

   Patient's weight: 250 lb

   ▶ **How many micrograms per kilogram per minute is the patient receiving?** _____

9. Order: Hydrea 30 mg/kg/day PO for ovarian carcinoma

   Patient's weight: 157 lb

   ▶ **How many grams per day is the patient receiving?** _____

(Practice Problems continue on page 194)

10. Order: Venoglobulin-S 0.01 mL/kg/min for treatment of
    immunodeficiency syndrome

    Patient's weight: 180 lb

    ▶ **Calculate the milliliters per hour to set
    the IV pump.** _____

11. Information obtained by the nurse: dopamine 400 mg in 250 mL
    D5W is infusing at 28 mL/hr.

    Patient's weight: 15 kg

    ▶ **How many micrograms per kilogram
    per minute is the patient receiving?** _____

12. Order: Inocor 3 mcg/kg/min IV for congestive heart failure

    Supply: Inocor 100 mg/100 mL of 0.9% NS

    Patient's weight: 160 lb

    ▶ **Calculate the milliliters per hour to set
    the IV pump.** _____

13. Order: Nipride 2 mcg/kg/min

    Supply: Nipride 50 mg/250 mL NS

    Patient's weight: 250 lb

    ▶ **Calculate the milliliters per hour to
    set the IV pump.** _____

14. Order: Nipride 1 mcg/kg/min IV for hypertensive crisis

    Supply: Nipride 50 mg/250 mL NS

    Patient's weight: 160 lb

    ▶ **Calculate the milliliters per hour to set
    the IV pump.**

15. Order: dopamine 2.5 mcg/kg/min IV for hypotension

    Supply: dopamine 400 mg/500 mL D5W

    Patient's weight: 65 kg

    ▶ **Calculate the milliliters per hour to set
    the IV pump.**

16. Information obtained by the nurse: Isuprel 2 mg in 500 mL D5W is
    infusing at 15 mL/hr.

    Child's weight: 20 kg

    ▶ **How many micrograms per kilogram
    per minute is the child receiving?** _____

17. Order: Intropin 5 mcg/kg/min IV for treatment of oliguria after shock

    Supply: Intropin 400 mg/500 mL NS

    Patient's weight: 70 kg

    ▶ **Calculate the milliliters per minute.** _____

18. Order: vancomycin 40 mg/kg/day IV in three divided doses for infection

    Supply: vancomycin 500-mg vial

    Nursing drug reference: Reconstitute each 500-mg vial with 10 mL sterile

    water and further dilute in 100 mL of 0.9% NS to infuse over 60 minutes.

    Child's weight: 20 lb

    ▶ **How many milligrams per day is the**
       child receiving? _____

    ▶ **How many milligrams per dose is the**
       child receiving? _____

    ▶ **How many milliliters will you draw from the vial**
       after reconstitution? _____

    ▶ **Calculate the milliliters per hour to set**
       the IV pump. _____

19. Order: gentamicin 2 mg/kg/dose IV every 8 hours for infection

    Supply: gentamicin 40-mg/mL vial

    Nursing drug reference: Further dilute in 50 mL NS and infuse over

    30 minutes.

    Child's weight: 40 kg

    ▶ **How many milligrams per dose is the**
       child receiving? _____

    ▶ **How many milliliters will you draw**
       from the vial? _____

    ▶ **Calculate the milliliters per hour to set**
       the IV pump. _____

(Practice Problems continue on page 196)

20. Order: Ancef 25 mg/kg/day IV every 8 hours for infection

    Supply: Ancef 500-mg vial

    Nursing drug reference: Reconstitute each 500-mg vial with 10 mL of sterile water and further dilute in 50 mL NS to infuse over 30 minutes.

    Child's weight: 25 kg

    ▶ **How many milligrams per day is the child receiving?** _____

    ▶ **How many milligrams per dose is the child receiving?** _____

    ▶ **How many milliliters will you draw from the vial after reconstitution?** _____

    ▶ **Calculate the milliliters per hour to set the IV pump.** _____

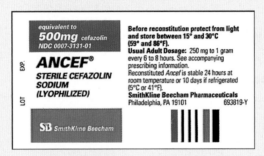

Courtesy of SmithKline Beecham Pharmaceuticals.

21. Order: Amikacin (Amikin) 15 mg/kg/day IV in 2 equally divided doses every 12 hours for 10 days for gram-negative bacterial infection

    Supply: Amikin 500 mg in 100 mL 0.9% Normal Saline to infuse over 60 minutes

    Patient's weight: 80 kg

    ▶ **How many milligrams per day is the patient receiving?** _____

    ▶ **How many milligrams per dose is the patient receiving?** _____

    ▶ **Calculate the milliliters per hour to set the IV pump.** _____

22. Order: dopamine (Intropin) 2 mcg/kg/minute IV for shock

    Supply: dopamine 200 mg/250 mL D5W

    Patient's weight: 175 lb

    ▶ **Calculate the milliliters per hour to set the IV pump.**

23. Order: epoetin (Procrit) 150 units/kg/day three times a week for

    chemotherapy-induced anemia

    Supply: Procrit 10,000 units/mL

    Patient's weight: 80 kg

    ▶ **How many milliliters per day will you give?** _____

24. Order: esmolol hydrochloride 500 mcg/kg/min for 1 minute then

    50 mcg/kg/min for 4 minutes for supraventricular tachycardia in atrial

    fibrillation. Repeat after 5 minutes if SVT continues.

    Supply: esmolol 2.5 g/250 mL D5W

    Patient's weight: 90 kg

    ▶ **Calculate the milliliters per hour to set the IV pump for the
    one minute administration.** _____

    ▶ **Calculate the milliliters per hour to set the IV pump for the
    four minute administration.** _____

25. Order: prednisone 0.1 mg/kg/day for chronic obstructive pulmonary

    disease.

    Supply: prednisone 5 mg/5 mL oral solution

    Child's weight: 35 kg

    ▶ **How many milliliter per day will you give?** _____

Practice Problems	**Comprehensive Practice Problems**

(See pages 213–215 for answers)

1. Order: digoxin 0.125 mg PO daily for congestive heart failure

   On hand: digoxin 0.25 mg/tablet

   ▶ **How many tablets will you give?** _____

2. Order: ascorbic acid 0.5 g PO daily for supplemental therapy

   On hand: ascorbic acid 500 mg/tablet

   ▶ **How many tablets will you give?** _____

3. Order: atropine gr 1/150 IM for on-call preanesthesia

   Supply: atropine 0.4 mg/mL

   ▶ **How many milliliters will you give?** _____

(Practice Problems continue on page 198)

4. Order: Mycostatin oral suspension 500,000 units swish-and-swallow for oral thrush

   On hand: Mycostatin 100,000 units/mL

   ▶ **How many teaspoons will you give?** _____

5. Order: Demerol 50 mg IM every 4 hours for pain

   Supply: Demerol 100 mg/mL

   ▶ **How many milliliters will you give?** _____

6. Order: vancomycin 2 mg/kg IV every 12 hours for infection

   Supply: vancomycin 500 mg/10 mL

   Patient's weight: 75 kg

   ▶ **How many milliliters will you give?** _____

7. Order: ampicillin 2 mg/kg PO every 8 hours for infection

   Supply: ampicillin 500 mg/5 mL

   Patient's weight: 100 lb

   ▶ **How many milliliters will you give?** _____

8. Order: 1000 mL D5W to infuse in 12 hours

   Drop factor: 15 gtt/mL

   ▶ **Calculate the number of drops per minute.** _____

9. Order: 500 mL D5W

   Drop factor: 15 gtt/mL

   Infusion rate: 21 gtt/min

   ▶ **Calculate the hours to infuse.** _____

10. Order: heparin 1500 units/hr

    Supply: 250-mL IV bag of D5W with 25,000 units of heparin

    ▶ **Calculate the milliliters per hour to set the IV pump.** _____

11. Order: 1000 mL NS IV

    Drop factor: 15 gtt/mL

    Infusion rate: 50 gtt/min

    ▶ **Calculate the hours to infuse.** _____

12. Order: regular insulin 8 units per hour IV for hyperglycemia

    Supply: 250 mL NS with 100 units of regular insulin

    ▶ **Calculate the milliliters per hour
    to set the IV pump.** _____

13. Order: 500 mL of 10% lipids to infuse in 8 hours

    Drop factor: 10 gtt/mL

    ▶ **Calculate the number of drops per minute.** _____

14. Order: KCl 2 mEq/100 mL of D5W for hypokalemia

    On hand: 20 mEq/10-mL vial

    Supply: 500 mL D5W

    ▶ **How many milliliters of KCl
    will you add to the IV bag?** _____

15. Order: aminophylline 44 mg/hr IV for bronchodilation

    Supply: 250 mL D5W with 1 g of aminophylline

    ▶ **Calculate the milliliters per hour
    to set the IV pump.** _____

16. Order: Dilaudid 140 mL/hr

    Supply: 1000 mL D5W/NS with 30 mg of Dilaudid

    ▶ **Calculate the milligrams per hour
    that the patient is receiving.** _____

17. Order: Staphcillin 750 mg IV every 4 hours for infection

    Supply: Staphcillin 6 g

    Nursing drug reference: Reconstitute with 8.6 mL of sterile water to yield

    500 mg/mL and further dilute in 100 mL of NS to infuse over 30 minutes.

    ▶ **How many milliliters will you draw from the vial after
    reconstitution?** _____

    ▶ **Calculate the milliliters per hour
    to set the IV pump.** _____

    ▶ **Calculate the drops per minute with
    a drop factor of 10 gtt/mL.** _____

(Practice Problems continue on page 200)

18. Order: Pipracil 1.5 g every 6 hours for uncomplicated urinary

    tract infection

    Supply: Pipracil 3-g vial

    Nursing drug reference: Reconstitute each 3-g vial with 5 mL of sterile

    water and further dilute in 50 mL of 0.9% NS to infuse over 20 minutes.

    ▶ **How many milliliters will you draw from the
    vial after reconstitution?** _____

    ▶ **Calculate the milliliters per hour
    to set the IV pump.** _____

    ▶ **Calculate the drops per minute with
    a drop factor of 20 gtt/mL.** _____

19. Order: dopamine 4 mcg/kg/min IV for decreased cardiac output

    Supply: 250 mL D5W with 400 mg of dopamine

    Patient's weight: 120 lb

    ▶ **Calculate the milliliters per hour
    to set the IV pump.** _____

20. Order: Nipride 0.8 mcg/kg/min IV for hypertension

    Supply: 500 mL D5W with 50 mg Nipride

    Patient's weight: 143 lb

    ▶ **Calculate the milliliters per hour
    to set the IV pump.** _____

21. Order: ampicillin (Principen) 500 mg PO every 6 hours for

    chronic infection

    Supply: 250 mg/5 mL

    ▶ **How many milliliters will you give?** _____

22. Order: atenolol (Tenormin) 50 mg PO per day for hypertension

    Supply: atenolol 100 mg tablets.

    ▶ **How many tablets will you give?** _____

23. Order: amiodarone (Cordarone IV) 150 mg IV over 10 minutes

    Supply: amiodarone 150 mg in 100 mL D5W

    ▶ **Calculate the milliliters per hour to set the
    IV pump.** _____

24. Order: azithromycin (Zithromax) 30 mg/kg PO once a day for
    three days for otitis media.

    Supply: azithromycin 100 mg/5 mL

    Child's weight: 15 kg

    ▶ **How many milliliters will you give?** _____

25. Order: amoxicillin 45 mg/kg/day in two divided doses for severe
    ear infection.

    Supply: amoxicillin 400 mg/5 mL

    Child's weight: 35 kg

    ▶ **How many milligrams per day is the
    child receiving?** _____

    ▶ **How many milligrams per dose is the
    child receiving?** _____

    ▶ **How many milliliters per dose will you give?** _____

ANSWER KEY FOR SECTION 2: PRACTICE PROBLEMS

One-Factor Practice Problems

1. Sequential method:

$$\frac{200 \text{ mg} \quad \boxed{\text{mL}} \quad 2}{100 \text{ mg} \quad 1} = 2 \text{ mL}$$

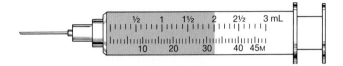

2. Sequential method:

$$\frac{30 \text{ mg} \quad \boxed{\text{tablet}} \quad 3}{30 \text{ mg} \quad 3} = 1 \text{ tablet}$$

3. Sequential method:

$$\frac{7.5 \text{ mg} \quad \boxed{\text{tablet}} \quad 7.5}{2.5 \text{ mg} \quad 2.5} = 3 \text{ tablets}$$

4. Sequential method:

$$\frac{160 \text{ mg} \quad 5 \text{ mL} \quad 1 \; \boxed{\text{tsp}} \quad 1}{160 \text{ mg} \quad 5 \text{ mL}} = 1 \text{ tsp}$$

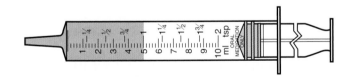

5. Sequential method:

$$\frac{0.5 \text{ mg} \quad \boxed{\text{tablet}} \quad 0.5}{1 \text{ mg} \quad 1} = 0.5 \text{ tablet}$$

6. Sequential method:

$$\frac{60 \text{ mg} \quad \boxed{\text{tablet}}}{60 \text{ mg}} = 1 \text{ tablet}$$

7. Sequential method:

$$\frac{0.25 \text{ mg} \quad \boxed{\text{tablet}} \quad 0.25}{0.125 \text{ mg} \quad 0.125} = 2 \text{ tablets}$$

8. Sequential method:

$$\frac{80 \text{ mg} \quad \boxed{\text{tablet}} \quad 8}{20 \text{ mg} \quad 2} = 4 \text{ tablets}$$

9. Random method:

$$\frac{10 \text{ mg} \quad \boxed{\text{mL}} \quad 1 \text{ gr} \quad 1 \times 1 \quad 1 \quad 1}{\frac{1}{8} \text{ gr} \quad 60 \text{ mg} \quad \frac{1}{8} \times \frac{6}{1} \quad \frac{6}{8} \quad 0.75} = \begin{array}{l} 1.33 \text{ or} \\ 1.3 \text{ mL} \end{array}$$

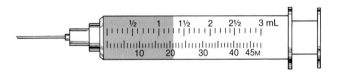

10. Random method:

$$\frac{100 \text{ mcg} \quad \boxed{\text{mL}} \quad 1 \text{ mg} \quad 1 \times 1 \quad 1}{0.4 \text{ mg} \quad 1000 \text{ mcg} \quad 0.4 \times 10 \quad 4} = \begin{array}{l} 0.25 \text{ or} \\ 0.3 \text{ mL} \end{array}$$

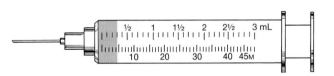

11. Sequential method:

$$\frac{80 \text{ mg} \quad 2 \; \boxed{\text{mL}} \quad 80 \times 2 \quad 160}{125 \text{ mg} \quad 125 \quad 125} = 1.28 \text{ or } 1.3 \text{ mL}$$

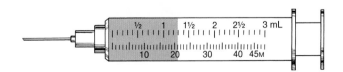

12. Sequential method:

$$\frac{2\theta \text{ g}}{} \left| \frac{15 \text{ (mL)}}{1\theta \text{ g}} \right| \frac{2 \times 15}{1} \left| \frac{30}{1} \right. = 30 \text{ mL}$$

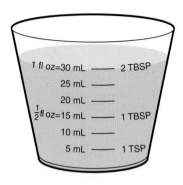

13. Sequential method:

$$\frac{5 \text{ mg}}{} \left| \frac{\text{(mL)}}{5 \text{ mg}} \right. = 1 \text{ mL}$$

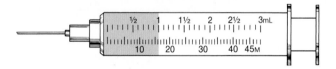

14. Sequential method:

$$\frac{250 \text{ mg}}{} \left| \frac{5 \text{ (mL)}}{125 \text{ mg}} \right| \frac{250 \times 5}{125} \left| \frac{1250}{125} \right. = 10 \text{ mL}$$

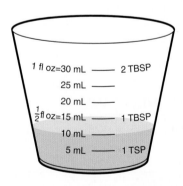

15. Sequential method:

$$\frac{200 \text{ mg}}{} \left| \frac{\text{(capsules)}}{100 \text{ mg}} \right| \frac{2}{1} = 2 \text{ capsules}$$

16. Sequential method:

$$\frac{10 \text{ mg}}{} \left| \frac{\text{(tablet)}}{5 \text{ mg}} \right| \frac{10}{5} = 2 \text{ tablets}$$

17. Sequential method:

$$\frac{3 \text{ mg}}{} \left| \frac{\text{(mL)}}{2 \text{ mg}} \right| \frac{3}{2} = 1.5 \text{ mL}$$

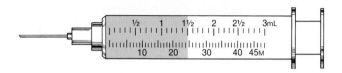

18. Sequential method:

$$\frac{400 \text{ mg}}{} \left| \frac{10.15 \text{ (mL)}}{325 \text{ mg}} \right| \frac{400 \times 10.15}{325} \left| \frac{4060}{325} \right. = \begin{matrix} 12.49 \text{ or} \\ 12.5 \text{ mL} \end{matrix}$$

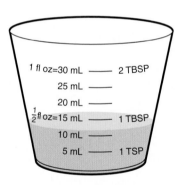

19. Random method:

$$\frac{1000 \text{ mg}}{} \left| \frac{2 \text{ (mL)}}{1 \text{ g}} \right| \frac{1 \text{ g}}{1000 \text{ mg}} \left| \frac{2 \times 1}{1} \right| \frac{2}{1} = 2 \text{ mL}$$

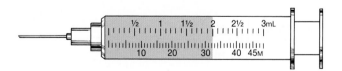

20. Sequential method:

$$\frac{10 \text{ mg}}{} \left| \frac{5 \text{ mL}}{5 \text{ mg}} \right| \frac{1 \text{ (tsp)}}{5 \text{ mL}} \left| \frac{10 \times 1}{5} \right| \frac{10}{5} = 2 \text{ tsp}$$

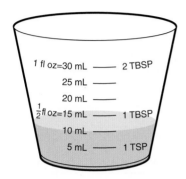

21. Random method:

$$\frac{0.25 \text{ mg}}{} \left| \frac{\text{(mL)}}{250 \text{ mcg}} \right| \frac{1000 \text{ mcg}}{1 \text{ mg}} \left| \frac{0.25 \times 100}{25 \times 1} \right| \frac{25}{25} = 1 \text{ mL}$$

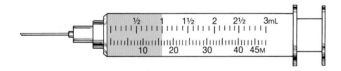

22. Sequential method:

$$\frac{500 \text{ mg}}{} \left| \frac{\text{(mL)}}{300 \text{ mg}} \right| \frac{5}{3} = 1.66 \text{ or } 1.7 \text{ mL}$$

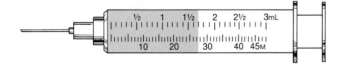

23. Sequential method:

$$\frac{2500 \text{ IU}}{} \left| \frac{0.2 \text{ (mL)}}{2500 \text{ IU}} \right| \frac{0.2}{} = 0.2 \text{ mL}$$

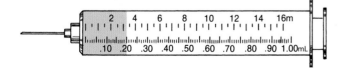

24. Sequential method:

$$\frac{200 \text{ mg}}{} \left| \frac{5 \text{ (mL)}}{50 \text{ mg}} \right| \frac{20 \times 5}{5} \left| \frac{100}{5} \right| = 20 \text{ mL}$$

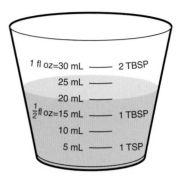

25. Sequential method:

$$\frac{300 \text{ mg}}{} \left| \frac{\text{(capsule)}}{150 \text{ mg}} \right| \frac{30}{15} = 2 \text{ capsules}$$

26. Sequential method:

$$\frac{500 \text{ mg}}{} \left| \frac{\text{(tablets)}}{500 \text{ mg}} \right| \frac{500}{500} = 1 \text{ tablet}$$

27. Sequential method:

$$\frac{0.25 \text{ mg}}{} \left| \frac{\text{(tablets)}}{0.125 \text{ mg}} \right| \frac{0.25}{0.125} = 2 \text{ tablets}$$

28. Sequential method:

$$\frac{25 \text{ mg}}{} \left| \frac{\text{(tablets)}}{50 \text{ mg}} \right| \frac{25}{50} = 0.5 \text{ tablet}$$

29. Sequential method:

$$\frac{5 \text{ mg}}{} \left| \frac{\text{(tablets)}}{2.5 \text{ mg}} \right| \frac{5}{2.5} = 2 \text{ tablets}$$

30. Sequential method:

$$\frac{0.5 \text{ mg}}{} \left| \frac{\text{(tablets)}}{0.25 \text{ mg}} \right| \frac{0.5}{0.25} = 2 \text{ tablets}$$

31. Sequential method:

$$\frac{150 \text{ mg} \quad | \quad \fbox{mL} \quad | \quad 15}{| \quad 400 \text{ mg} \quad | \quad 40} = 0.375 \text{ or } 0.4 \text{ mL}$$

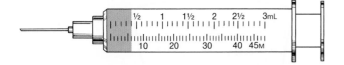

32. Sequential method:

$$\frac{600 \text{ mg} \quad | \quad \fbox{tablets} \quad | \quad 6}{| \quad 300 \text{ mg} \quad | \quad 3} = 2 \text{ tablets}$$

33. Sequential method:

$$\frac{60 \text{ mg} \quad | \quad 5 \fbox{mL} \quad | \quad 6 \times 5 \quad | \quad 30}{| \quad 20 \text{ mg} \quad | \quad 2 \quad | \quad 2} = 15 \text{ mL}$$

34. Sequential method:

$$\frac{600 \text{ mg} \quad | \quad \fbox{tablet} \quad | \quad 6}{| \quad 300 \text{ mg} \quad | \quad 3} = 2 \text{ tablets}$$

35. Sequential method:

$$\frac{100 \text{ mg} \quad | \quad \fbox{mL} \quad | \quad 10}{| \quad 10 \text{ mg} \quad | \quad 1} = 10 \text{ mL}$$

Two-Factor Practice Problems

1. Random method:

$$\frac{25 \text{ mcg} \quad | \quad 2.5 \fbox{mL} \quad | \quad 1 \text{ kg} \quad | \quad 1 \text{ mg} \quad | \quad 25 \text{ lb}}{\text{kg} \quad | \quad 0.125 \text{ mg} \quad | \quad 2.2 \text{ lb} \quad | \quad 1000 \text{ mcg} \quad |} = \text{ mL}$$

$$\frac{25 \times 2.5 \times 1 \times 1 \times 25 \quad | \quad 1562.5}{0.125 \times 2.2 \times 1000 \quad | \quad 275} = 5.68 \text{ or } 5.7 \text{ mL}$$

2. Sequential method:

$$\frac{0.02 \text{ mg} \quad | \quad \fbox{mL} \quad | \quad 1 \text{ kg} \quad | \quad 35 \text{ lb}}{\text{kg} \quad | \quad 0.1 \text{ mg} \quad | \quad 2.2 \text{ lb} \quad |} \frac{0.02 \times 1 \times 35 \quad | \quad 0.7}{0.1 \times 2.2 \quad | \quad 0.22} = \frac{3.18 \text{ or}}{3.2 \text{ mL}}$$

3. Random method:

$$\frac{2 \text{ mg} \quad | \quad 500 \fbox{mL} \quad | \quad 1 \text{ g} \quad | \quad 60 \text{ min} \quad | \quad 5 \times 6 \quad | \quad 30}{\text{min} \quad | \quad 2 \text{ g} \quad | \quad 1000 \text{ mg} \quad | \quad 1 \fbox{hr} \quad | \quad 1 \quad | \quad 1} = \frac{30 \text{ mL}}{\text{hr}}$$

4. Sequential method:

$$\frac{1.5 \text{ g} \quad | \quad 10 \fbox{mL} \quad | \quad 1.5 \times 10 \quad | \quad 15}{| \quad 1 \text{ g} \quad | \quad 1 \quad | \quad 1} = 15 \text{ mL}$$

5. Sequential method:

$$\frac{1 \text{ mg} \quad | \quad \fbox{mL} \quad | \quad 1 \text{ kg} \quad | \quad 94 \text{ lb} \quad | \quad 1 \times 1 \times 94 \quad | \quad 94}{\text{kg} \quad | \quad 40 \text{ mg} \quad | \quad 2.2 \text{ lb} \quad | \quad | \quad 40 \times 2.2 \quad | \quad 88} = \frac{1.068 \text{ or}}{1.1 \text{ mL}}$$

6. Sequential method:

$$\frac{15 \text{ mg} \quad | \quad 500 \fbox{mL} \quad | \quad 15 \times 5 \quad | \quad 75}{\fbox{hr} \quad | \quad 300 \text{ mg} \quad | \quad 3 \quad | \quad 3} = \frac{25 \text{ mL}}{\text{hr}}$$

7. Sequential method:

$$\frac{25 \text{ mL} \quad | \quad 50 \fbox{mg} \quad | \quad 5}{\fbox{hr} \quad | \quad 250 \text{ mL} \quad |} = \frac{5 \text{ mg}}{\text{hr}}$$

8. Sequential method:

$$\frac{10 \text{ mEq} \quad | \quad 20 \fbox{mL} \quad | \quad 10}{| \quad 20 \text{ mEq} \quad |} = 10 \text{ mL}$$

9. Sequential method:

$$\frac{3 \text{ mL} \quad | \quad 50 \text{ mg} \quad | \quad 1000 \fbox{mcg} \quad | \quad 1 \text{ hr} \quad | \quad 3 \times 10 \quad | \quad 30}{\text{hr} \quad | \quad 500 \text{ mL} \quad | \quad 1 \text{ mg} \quad | \quad 60 \fbox{min} \quad | \quad 6 \quad | \quad 6} = \frac{5 \text{ mcg}}{\text{min}}$$

10. Sequential method:

$$\frac{100 \text{ mL} \quad | \quad 10 \fbox{mEq} \quad | \quad 1}{\fbox{hr} \quad | \quad 1000 \text{ mL} \quad |} = \frac{1 \text{ mEq}}{\text{hr}}$$

11. Sequential method:

$$\frac{250 \text{ mL} \quad | \quad 20 \fbox{gtt} \quad | \quad 1 \text{ hr} \quad | \quad 250 \times 2 \times 1 \quad | \quad 500}{\text{hr} \quad | \quad \text{mL} \quad | \quad 60 \fbox{min} \quad | \quad 6 \quad | \quad 6} = \frac{83.3 \text{ or } 83 \text{ gtt}}{\text{min}}$$

12. Sequential method:

$$\frac{750 \text{ mL}}{5 \text{ hr}} \left| \frac{10 \text{ gtt}}{\text{mL}} \right| \frac{1 \text{ hr}}{60 \text{ min}} \left| \frac{750 \times 1 \times 1}{5 \times 6} \right| \frac{750}{30} = \frac{25 \text{ gtt}}{\text{min}}$$

13. Sequential method:

$$\frac{500 \text{ mL}}{8 \text{ hr}} \left| \frac{60 \text{ gtt}}{\text{mL}} \right| \frac{1 \text{ hr}}{60 \text{ min}} \left| \frac{500 \times 1}{8} \right| \frac{500}{8} = \frac{62.5 \text{ or } 63 \text{ gtt}}{\text{min}}$$

14. Sequential method:

$$\frac{750 \text{ mL}}{} \left| \frac{15 \text{ gtt}}{\text{mL}} \right| \frac{\text{min}}{18 \text{ gtt}} \left| \frac{1 \text{ hr}}{60 \text{ min}} \right| \frac{750 \times 15 \times 1}{18 \times 60} \left| \frac{11250}{1080} \right| = \frac{10.41 \text{ or}}{10 \text{ hr}}$$

15. Sequential method:

$$\frac{250 \text{ mL}}{} \left| \frac{15 \text{ gtt}}{\text{mL}} \right| \frac{\text{min}}{50 \text{ gtt}} \left| \frac{1 \text{ hr}}{60 \text{ min}} \right| \frac{25 \times 15 \times 1}{50 \times 6} \left| \frac{375}{300} \right| = \frac{1.25 \text{ or}}{1 \text{ hr}}$$

16. Sequential method:

$$\frac{1000 \text{ mL}}{} \left| \frac{15 \text{ gtt}}{\text{mL}} \right| \frac{\text{min}}{25 \text{ gtt}} \left| \frac{1 \text{ hr}}{60 \text{ min}} \right| \frac{100 \times 15 \times 1}{25 \times 6} \left| \frac{1500}{150} \right| = 10 \text{ hr}$$

17. How many milliliters will you draw from the vial after reconstitution?
Sequential method:

$$\frac{1.25 \text{ g}}{} \left| \frac{10 \text{ mL}}{1 \text{ g}} \right| \frac{1.25 \times 10}{1} \left| \frac{12.5}{1} \right| = 12.5 \text{ mL}$$

Calculate the milliliters per hour to set the IV pump.
Sequential method:

$$\frac{112.5 \text{ mL}}{\text{hr}} = 112.5 \text{ or } \frac{113 \text{ mL}}{\text{hr}}$$

Calculate the drops per minute with a drop factor of 10 gtt/mL.
Sequential method:

$$\frac{112.5 \text{ mL}}{\text{hr}} \left| \frac{10 \text{ gtt}}{\text{mL}} \right| \frac{1 \text{ hr}}{60 \text{ min}} \left| \frac{112.5 \times 1 \times 1}{6} \right| \frac{112.5}{6} = \frac{18.75 \text{ or } 19 \text{ gtt}}{\text{min}}$$

18. How many milliliters will you draw from the vial after reconstitution?
Sequential method:

$$\frac{275 \text{ mg}}{} \left| \frac{10 \text{ mL}}{500 \text{ mg}} \right| \frac{275 \times 1}{50} \left| \frac{275}{50} \right| = 5.5 \text{ mL}$$

Calculate the milliliters per hour to set the IV pump.
Sequential method:

$$\frac{255.5 \text{ mL}}{\text{hr}} = 255.5 \text{ or } \frac{256 \text{ mL}}{\text{hr}}$$

Calculate the drops per minute with a drop factor of 10 gtt/mL.
Sequential method:

$$\frac{255.5 \text{ mL}}{\text{hr}} \left| \frac{10 \text{ gtt}}{\text{mL}} \right| \frac{1 \text{ hr}}{60 \text{ min}} \left| \frac{255.5 \times 1 \times 1}{6} \right| \frac{255.5}{6} = \frac{42.5 \text{ or } 43 \text{ gtt}}{\text{min}}$$

19. How many milliliters will you draw from the vial after reconstitution?
Random method:

$$\frac{450 \text{ mg}}{} \left| \frac{10 \text{ mL}}{1 \text{ g}} \right| \frac{1 \text{ g}}{1000 \text{ mg}} \left| \frac{45 \times 1}{10} \right| \frac{45}{10} = 4.5 \text{ mL}$$

Calculate the milliliters per hour to set the IV pump.
Sequential method:

$$\frac{104.5 \text{ mL}}{30 \text{ min}} \left| \frac{60 \text{ min}}{1 \text{ hr}} \right| \frac{104.5 \times 6}{3 \times 1} \left| \frac{627}{3} \right| = \frac{209 \text{ mL}}{\text{hr}}$$

Calculate the drops per minute with a drop factor of 10 gtt/mL.
Sequential method:

$$\frac{104.5 \text{ mL}}{30 \text{ min}} \left| \frac{10 \text{ gtt}}{\text{mL}} \right| \frac{104.5 \times 1}{3} \left| \frac{104.5}{3} \right| = \frac{34.8 \text{ or } 35 \text{ gtt}}{\text{min}}$$

20. How many milliliters will you draw from the vial?
Sequential method:

$$\frac{23 \ \text{mg}}{} \ \left|\ \frac{\text{mL}}{40 \ \text{mg}} \ \right| \ \frac{23}{40} = 0.57 \ \text{or} \ 0.6 \ \text{mL}$$

Calculate the milliliters per hour to set the IV pump.
Sequential method:

$$\frac{100.6 \ \text{mL}}{\text{hr}} = 100.6 \ \text{or} \ \frac{101 \ \text{mL}}{\text{hr}}$$

Calculate the drops per minute with a drop factor of 15 gtt/mL.

$$\frac{100.6 \ \text{mL}}{\text{hr}} \ \left|\ \frac{15 \ \text{gtt}}{\text{mL}} \ \right| \ \frac{1 \ \text{hr}}{60 \ \text{min}} \ \left|\ \frac{100.6 \times 15 \times 1}{60} \ \right| \ \frac{1509}{60} = 25.15 \ \text{or} \ 25 \ \frac{\text{gtt}}{\text{min}}$$

21. Sequential method:

$$\frac{0.56 \ \text{mg}}{\text{kg}} \ \left|\ \frac{18 \ \text{kg}}{} \ \right| \ \frac{5 \ \text{mL}}{10 \ \text{mg}} \ \left|\ \frac{0.56 \times 18 \times 5}{10} \ \right| \ \frac{50.4}{10} = 5.04 \ \text{or} \ 5 \ \text{mL}$$

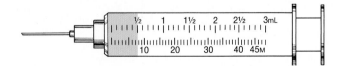

22. Random method:

$$\frac{30 \ \text{g}}{\text{day}} \ \left|\ \frac{\text{day}}{4 \ \text{doses}} \ \right| \ \frac{\text{packet}}{5 \ \text{g}} \ \left|\ \frac{30}{4 \times 5} \ \right| \ \frac{30}{20} = 1.5 \ \frac{\text{packet}}{\text{dose}}$$

23. Random method:

$$\frac{10 \ \text{mcg}}{\text{kg}} \ \left|\ \frac{2 \ \text{mL}}{2 \ \text{mg}} \ \right| \ \frac{50 \ \text{kg}}{} \ \left|\ \frac{1 \ \text{mg}}{1000 \ \text{mcg}} \ \right| \ \frac{1 \times 2 \times 5 \times 1}{2 \times 10} \ \left|\ \frac{10}{20} \ \right| = 0.5 \ \text{mL}$$

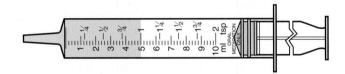

24. Sequential method:

$$\frac{1600 \ \text{mg}}{\text{day}} \ \left|\ \frac{\text{tablets}}{800 \ \text{mg}} \ \right| \ \frac{\text{day}}{2 \ \text{doses}} \ \left|\ \frac{16}{8 \times 2} \ \right| \ \frac{16}{16} = 1 \ \frac{\text{tablet}}{\text{dose}}$$

25. Random method:

$$\frac{1 \ \text{g}}{\text{day}} \ \left|\ \frac{\text{mL}}{100 \ \text{mg}} \ \right| \ \frac{1000 \ \text{mg}}{1 \ \text{g}} \ \left|\ \frac{\text{day}}{3 \ \text{doses}} \ \right| \ \frac{10}{1 \times 3} \ \left|\ \frac{10}{} \ \right| = \frac{3.33}{\text{or} \ 3} \ \frac{\text{mL}}{\text{dose}}$$

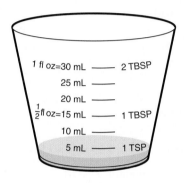

26. Sequential method:

$$\frac{4 \ \text{mg}}{\text{kg}} \ \left|\ \frac{\text{mL}}{10 \ \text{mg}} \ \right| \ \frac{20 \ \text{kg}}{} \ \left|\ \frac{4 \times 2}{1} \ \right| \ \frac{8}{1} = 8 \ \text{mL}$$

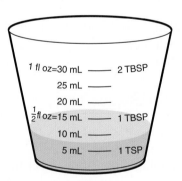

27. Sequential method:

$$\frac{0.15 \ \text{mg}}{\text{kg}} \ \left|\ \frac{\text{mL}}{2 \ \text{mg}} \ \right| \ \frac{1 \ \text{kg}}{2.2 \ \text{lb}} \ \left|\ \frac{160 \ \text{lb}}{} \ \right| \ \frac{0.15 \times 1 \times 160}{2 \times 2.2} \ \left|\ \frac{24}{4.4} \ \right| = \frac{5.45 \ \text{or}}{5.5 \ \text{mL}}$$

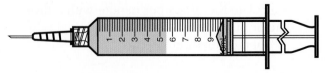

28. Sequential method:

$$\frac{2 \ \text{mg}}{\text{kg}} \left| \frac{\text{tablets}}{150 \ \text{mg}} \right| \frac{40 \ \text{kg}}{} \left| \frac{2 \times 4}{15} \right| \frac{8}{15} = \frac{0.533 \ \text{or}}{0.5 \ \text{tablet}}$$

29. Sequential method:

$$\frac{20 \ \text{mg}}{\text{kg}} \left| \frac{\text{tablet}}{400 \ \text{mg}} \right| \frac{1 \ \text{kg}}{2.2 \ \text{lb}} \left| \frac{20 \ \text{lb}}{} \right| \frac{2 \times 1 \times 2}{4 \times 2.2} \left| \frac{4}{8.8} \right. = \frac{0.45 \ \text{or}}{0.5 \ \text{tablet}}$$

30. Sequential method:

$$\frac{450 \ \text{mg}}{\text{day}} \left| \frac{\text{tablet}}{150 \ \text{mg}} \right| \frac{\text{day}}{3 \ \text{doses}} \left| \frac{45}{15 \times 3} \right| \frac{45}{45} = \frac{1 \ \text{tablet}}{\text{dose}}$$

31. Random method:

$$\frac{2.4 \ \text{g}}{\text{day}} \left| \frac{\text{tablet}}{300 \ \text{mg}} \right| \frac{\text{day}}{4 \ \text{doses}} \left| \frac{1000 \ \text{mg}}{1 \ \text{g}} \right| \frac{2.4 \times 10}{3 \times 4 \times 1} \left| \frac{24}{12} \right. = \frac{2 \ \text{tablets}}{\text{dose}}$$

32. Sequential method:

$$\frac{500 \ \text{mg}}{\text{day}} \left| \frac{8 \ \text{mL}}{750 \ \text{mg}} \right| \frac{\text{day}}{2 \ \text{doses}} \left| \frac{50 \times 8}{75 \times 2} \right| \frac{400}{150} = \frac{2.666 \ \text{or}}{\frac{2.7 \ \text{mL}}{\text{dose}}}$$

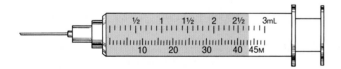

33. Random method:

$$\frac{1000 \ \text{mg}}{\text{day}} \left| \frac{20 \ \text{mL}}{2 \ \text{g}} \right| \frac{1 \ \text{g}}{1000 \ \text{mg}} \left| \frac{\text{day}}{2 \ \text{doses}} \right| \frac{20 \times 1}{2 \times 2} \left| \frac{20}{4} \right. = \frac{5 \ \text{mL}}{\text{dose}}$$

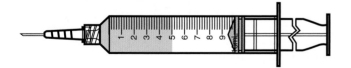

34. Sequential method:

$$\frac{150 \ \text{mg}}{2.2 \ \text{lb}/5 \ \text{doses}} \left| \frac{1 \ \text{tsp}}{500 \ \text{mg}} \right| \frac{2.2 \ \text{lb}}{1 \ \text{kg}} \left| \frac{30 \ \text{kg}}{} \right| \frac{5 \ \text{mL}}{1 \ \text{tsp}} = \frac{\text{mL}}{\text{dose}}$$

$$\frac{15 \times 3}{5 \times 1} \left| \frac{45}{5} \right. = \frac{9 \ \text{mL}}{\text{dose}}$$

35. Sequential method:

$$\frac{8 \ \text{mg}}{\text{kg}} \left| \frac{\text{mL}}{20 \ \text{mg}} \right| \frac{40 \ \text{kg}}{} \left| \frac{8 \times 4}{2} \right| \frac{32}{2} = 16 \ \text{mL}$$

Three-Factor Practice Problems

1. How many milliliters per day will you give?
   Sequential method:

$$\frac{40 \ \text{mg}}{\text{kg/day}} \left| \frac{5 \ \text{mL}}{300 \ \text{mg}} \right| \frac{60 \ \text{kg}}{} \left| \frac{4 \times 5 \times 6}{3} \right| \frac{120}{3} = \frac{40 \ \text{mL}}{\text{day}}$$

   How many milliliters per dose will you give?
   Sequential method:

$$\frac{40 \ \text{mg}}{\text{kg/day}} \left| \frac{5 \ \text{mL}}{300 \ \text{mg}} \right| \frac{60 \ \text{kg}}{} \left| \frac{\text{day}}{4 \ \text{doses}} \right| \frac{4 \times 5 \times 6}{3 \times 4} \left| \frac{120}{12} \right. = \frac{10 \ \text{mL}}{\text{dose}}$$

2. Sequential method:

$$\frac{4 \ \text{mg}}{\text{kg/day}} \left| \frac{\text{mL}}{10 \ \text{mg}} \right| \frac{1 \ \text{kg}}{2.2 \ \text{lb}} \left| \frac{60 \ \text{lb}}{} \right| \frac{4 \times 1 \times 6}{1 \times 2.2} \left| \frac{24}{2.2} \right. = \frac{10.9 \ \text{or} \ 11 \ \text{mL}}{\text{day}}$$

3. How many milliliters per day will you give?
   Sequential method:

$$\frac{30 \ \text{mg}}{\text{kg/day}} \left| \frac{2 \ \text{mL}}{300 \ \text{mg}} \right| \frac{50 \ \text{kg}}{} \left| \frac{2 \times 5}{} \right| \frac{10}{} = \frac{10 \ \text{mL}}{\text{day}}$$

   How many milliliters per dose will you give?
   Sequential method:

$$\frac{30 \ \text{mg}}{\text{kg/day}} \left| \frac{2 \ \text{mL}}{300 \ \text{mg}} \right| \frac{50 \ \text{kg}}{} \left| \frac{\text{day}}{3 \ \text{doses}} \right| \frac{2 \times 5}{3} \left| \frac{10}{3} \right. = \frac{3.33 \ \text{or} \ 3.3 \ \text{mL}}{\text{dose}}$$

4. Sequential method:

$$\frac{0.575 \text{ mL}}{\text{dose}} \left| \frac{40 \text{ (mg)}}{\text{mL}} \right| \frac{2.2 \text{ lb}}{1 \text{ (kg)}} \left| \frac{}{45 \text{ lb}} \right| \frac{3 \text{ doses}}{\text{(day)}} = \frac{\text{mg}}{\text{kg/day}}$$

$$\frac{0.575 \times 40 \times 2.2 \times 3}{1 \times 45} \left| \frac{151.8}{45} = \frac{3.37 \text{ or } 3.4}{} \frac{\text{mg}}{\text{kg/day}} \right.$$

5. Sequential method:

$$\frac{0.125 \text{ mL}}{\text{dose}} \left| \frac{50 \text{ (mg)}}{\text{mL}} \right| \frac{2.2 \text{ lb}}{1 \text{ (kg)}} \left| \frac{}{20 \text{ lb}} \right| \frac{3 \text{ doses}}{\text{(day)}} = \frac{\text{mg}}{\text{kg/day}}$$

$$\frac{0.125 \times 5 \times 2.2 \times 3}{1 \times 2} \left| \frac{4.125}{2} = \frac{2.06 \text{ or } 2.1}{} \frac{\text{mg}}{\text{kg/day}} \right.$$

6. How many milliliters will you draw from the vial?
   Sequential method:

$$\frac{400 \text{ mg}}{} \left| \frac{10 \text{ (mL)}}{400 \text{ mg}} \right| \frac{10}{} = 10 \text{ mL}$$

   Calculate the milliliters per hour to set the IV pump.
   Random method:

$$\frac{5 \text{ mcg}}{\text{kg/min}} \left| \frac{260 \text{ (mL)}}{400 \text{ mg}} \right| \frac{1 \text{ mg}}{1000 \text{ mcg}} \left| \frac{1 \text{ kg}}{2.2 \text{ lb}} \right| \frac{110 \text{ lb}}{} \left| \frac{60 \text{ min}}{1 \text{ (hr)}} \right| = \frac{\text{mL}}{\text{hr}}$$

$$\frac{5 \times 26 \times 1 \times 11 \times 6}{4 \times 100 \times 2.2} \left| \frac{8580}{880} = \frac{9.75 \text{ or } 9.8 \text{ mL}}{\text{hr}} \right.$$

7. Random method:

$$\frac{0.8 \text{ mcg}}{\text{kg/min}} \left| \frac{500 \text{ (mL)}}{50 \text{ mg}} \right| \frac{1 \text{ mg}}{1000 \text{ mcg}} \left| \frac{1 \text{ kg}}{2.2 \text{ lb}} \right| \frac{60 \text{ min}}{1 \text{ (hr)}} \left| \frac{143 \text{ lb}}{} \right| = \frac{\text{mL}}{\text{hr}}$$

$$\frac{0.8 \times 5 \times 1 \times 6 \times 143}{5 \times 10 \times 2.2} \left| \frac{3432}{110} = \frac{31.2 \text{ mL}}{\text{hr}} \right.$$

8. Sequential method:

$$\frac{68 \text{ mL}}{\text{hr}} \left| \frac{50 \text{ mg}}{250 \text{ mL}} \right| \frac{1 \text{ hr}}{60 \text{ (min)}} \left| \frac{2.2 \text{ lb}}{1 \text{ (kg)}} \right| \frac{1000 \text{ (mcg)}}{1 \text{ mg}} \left| \frac{}{250 \text{ lb}} \right| = \frac{\text{mcg}}{\text{kg/min}}$$

$$\frac{68 \times 5 \times 1 \times 2.2 \times 10}{25 \times 6 \times 1 \times 1 \times 25} \left| \frac{7480}{3750} = \frac{1.99 \text{ or } 2}{} \frac{\text{mcg}}{\text{kg/min}} \right.$$

9. Random method:

$$\frac{30 \text{ mg}}{\text{kg (day)}} \left| \frac{1 \text{ kg}}{2.2 \text{ lb}} \right| \frac{157 \text{ lb}}{} \left| \frac{1 \text{ (g)}}{1000 \text{ mg}} \right| \frac{3 \times 1 \times 157 \times 1}{2.2 \times 100} \left| \frac{471}{220} = \frac{2.14 \text{ or } 2.1}{} \frac{\text{g}}{\text{day}} \right.$$

10. Random method:

$$\frac{0.01 \text{ (mL)}}{\text{kg/min}} \left| \frac{1 \text{ kg}}{2.2 \text{ lb}} \right| \frac{180 \text{ lb}}{} \left| \frac{60 \text{ min}}{1 \text{ (hr)}} \right| \frac{0.01 \times 1 \times 180 \times 60}{2.2 \times 1}$$

$$\frac{108}{2.2} = \frac{49.09 \text{ or } 49.1 \text{ mL}}{\text{hr}}$$

11. Random method:

$$\frac{28 \text{ mL}}{\text{hr}} \left| \frac{400 \text{ mg}}{250 \text{ mL}} \right| \frac{}{15 \text{ (kg)}} \left| \frac{1 \text{ hr}}{60 \text{ (min)}} \right| \frac{1000 \text{ (mcg)}}{1 \text{ mg}} = \frac{\text{mcg}}{\text{kg/min}}$$

$$\frac{28 \times 4 \times 1 \times 1000}{25 \times 15 \times 6 \times 1} \left| \frac{112,000}{2250} = \frac{49.77 \text{ or } 49.8}{} \frac{\text{mcg}}{\text{kg/min}} \right.$$

12. Random method:

$$\frac{3 \text{ mcg}}{\text{kg/min}} \left| \frac{100 \text{ (mL)}}{100 \text{ mg}} \right| \frac{1 \text{ kg}}{2.2 \text{ lb}} \left| \frac{60 \text{ min}}{1 \text{ (hr)}} \right| \frac{160 \text{ lb}}{} \left| \frac{1 \text{ mg}}{1000 \text{ mcg}} \right| = \frac{\text{mL}}{\text{hr}}$$

$$\frac{3 \times 1 \times 6 \times 16 \times 1}{2.2 \times 1 \times 10} \left| \frac{288}{22} = \frac{13.09 \text{ or } 13.1 \text{mL}}{\text{hr}} \right.$$

13. Random method:

$$\frac{2 \text{ mcg}}{\text{kg/min}} \left| \frac{250 \text{ (mL)}}{50 \text{ mg}} \right| \frac{1 \text{ kg}}{2.2 \text{ lb}} \left| \frac{250 \text{ lb}}{} \right| \frac{1 \text{ mg}}{1000 \text{ mcg}} \left| \frac{60 \text{ min}}{1 \text{ (hr)}} \right|$$

$$\frac{2 \times 25 \times 1 \times 25 \times 6}{5 \times 2.2 \times 10} \left| \frac{7500}{110} = 68.1 \text{ or } \frac{68}{} \frac{\text{mL}}{\text{hr}} \right.$$

14. Random method:

$$\frac{1 \; \cancel{mcg}}{\cancel{kg/min}} \left| \frac{250 \; \cancel{mL}}{50 \; mg} \right| \frac{\cancel{1 \; kg}}{2.2 \; \cancel{lb}} \left| \frac{60 \; \cancel{min}}{1 \; \cancel{hr}} \right| \frac{160 \; \cancel{lb}}{} \left| \frac{\cancel{1 \; mg}}{1000 \; \cancel{mcg}} \right. = \frac{mL}{hr}$$

$$\frac{1 \times 25 \times 6 \times 16}{50 \times 2.2} \left| \frac{2400}{110} \right. = 21.81 \text{ or } 21.8 \; \frac{mL}{hr}$$

15. Random method:

$$\frac{2.5 \; \cancel{mcg}}{\cancel{kg/min}} \left| \frac{500 \; \cancel{mL}}{400 \; mg} \right| \frac{65 \; \cancel{kg}}{} \left| \frac{60 \; \cancel{min}}{1 \; \cancel{hr}} \right| \frac{1 \; \cancel{mg}}{1000 \; \cancel{mcg}} = \frac{mL}{hr}$$

$$\frac{2.5 \times 5 \times 65 \times 6 \times 1}{4 \times 1 \times 100} \left| \frac{4875}{400} \right. = 12.18 \text{ or } 12.2 \; \frac{mL}{hr}$$

16. Random method:

$$\frac{15 \; \cancel{mL}}{\cancel{hr}} \left| \frac{2 \; \cancel{mg}}{500 \; \cancel{mL}} \right| \frac{1 \; \cancel{hr}}{60 \; \cancel{min}} \left| \frac{}{20 \; \cancel{kg}} \right| \frac{1000 \; \cancel{mcg}}{1 \; \cancel{mg}} = \frac{mcg}{kg/min}$$

$$\frac{15 \times 2 \times 1 \times 1}{5 \times 6 \times 20 \times 1} \left| \frac{30}{600} \right. = 0.05 \; \frac{mcg}{kg/min}$$

17. Random method:

$$\frac{5 \; \cancel{mcg}}{\cancel{kg/min}} \left| \frac{500 \; \cancel{mL}}{400 \; mg} \right| \frac{70 \; \cancel{kg}}{} \left| \frac{1 \; \cancel{mg}}{1000 \; \cancel{mcg}} \right. = \frac{mL}{min}$$

$$\frac{5 \times 5 \times 7 \times 1}{4 \times 100} \left| \frac{175}{400} \right. = 0.4375 \text{ or } 0.44 \; \frac{mL}{min}$$

18. How many milligrams per day is the child receiving?
    Sequential method:

$$\frac{40 \; \cancel{mg}}{\cancel{kg/day}} \left| \frac{1 \; \cancel{kg}}{2.2 \; \cancel{lb}} \right| \frac{20 \; \cancel{lb}}{} \left| \frac{40 \times 1 \times 20}{2.2} \right| \frac{800}{2.2} = 363.63 \text{ or } 363.6 \; \frac{mg}{day}$$

How many milligrams per dose is the child receiving?
Sequential method:

$$\frac{363.6 \; \cancel{mg}}{\cancel{day}} \left| \frac{\cancel{day}}{3 \; \cancel{doses}} \right| \frac{363.6}{3} = 121.2 \; \frac{mg}{dose}$$

How many milliliters will you draw from the vial after reconstitution?
Sequential method:

$$\frac{121.2 \; \cancel{mg}}{} \left| \frac{10 \; \cancel{mL}}{500 \; \cancel{mg}} \right| \frac{121.2 \times 10}{500} \left| \frac{1212}{500} \right. = 2.424 \text{ or } 2.4 \; mL$$

Calculate the milliliters per hour to set the IV pump.
Sequential method:

$$\frac{102.4 \; \cancel{mL}}{60 \; \cancel{min}} \left| \frac{60 \; \cancel{min}}{1 \; \cancel{hr}} \right| \frac{102.4}{1} = 102.4 \; \frac{mL}{hr}$$

19. How many milligrams per dose is the child receiving?
    Random method:

$$\frac{2 \; \cancel{mg}}{\cancel{kg/dose}} \left| \frac{40 \; \cancel{kg}}{} \right| \frac{2 \times 40}{} \left| \frac{80}{} \right. = 80 \; \frac{mg}{dose}$$

How many milliliters will you draw from the vial?
Sequential method:

$$\frac{80 \; \cancel{mg}}{} \left| \frac{\cancel{mL}}{40 \; \cancel{mg}} \right| \frac{8}{4} = 2 \; mL$$

Calculate the milliliters per hour to set the IV pump.
Sequential method:

$$\frac{52 \; \cancel{mL}}{30 \; \cancel{min}} \left| \frac{60 \; \cancel{min}}{1 \; \cancel{hr}} \right| \frac{52 \times 6}{3 \times 1} \left| \frac{312}{3} \right. = 104 \; \frac{mL}{hr}$$

20. How many milligrams per day is the child receiving?
Sequential method:

$$\frac{25 \text{ (mg)}}{\text{kg/(day)}} \left| \frac{25 \text{ kg}}{} \right| \frac{25 \times 25}{} \left| \frac{625}{} \right| = \frac{625 \text{ mg}}{\text{day}}$$

How many milligrams per dose is the child receiving?
Sequential method:

$$\frac{625 \text{ (mg)}}{\text{day}} \left| \frac{\text{day}}{3 \text{ (doses)}} \right| \frac{625}{3} = 208.33 \text{ or } 208.3 \frac{\text{mg}}{\text{dose}}$$

How many milliliters will you draw from the vial after reconstitution?
Sequential method:

$$\frac{208.3 \text{ mg}}{} \left| \frac{10 \text{ (mL)}}{500 \text{ mg}} \right| \frac{208.3 \times 1}{50} \left| \frac{208.3}{50} \right| = 4.166 \text{ or } 4.2 \text{ mL}$$

Calculate the milliliters per hour to set the IV pump.
Sequential method:

$$\frac{54.2 \text{ (mL)}}{30 \text{ min}} \left| \frac{60 \text{ min}}{1 \text{ (hr)}} \right| \frac{54.2 \times 6}{3 \times 1} \left| \frac{325.2}{3} \right| = 108.4 \frac{\text{mL}}{\text{hr}}$$

21. Sequential method:
How many milligrams per day is the patient receiving?

$$\frac{15 \text{ (mg)}}{\text{kg/ (day)}} \left| \frac{80 \text{ kg}}{} \right| \frac{15 \times 80}{} \left| \frac{1200}{} \right| = 1200 \frac{\text{mg}}{\text{day}}$$

How many milligrams per dose is the patient receiving?

$$\frac{1200 \text{ (mg)}}{\text{day}} \left| \frac{\text{day}}{2 \text{ (doses)}} \right| \frac{1200}{2} = 600 \frac{\text{mg}}{\text{dose}}$$

Calculate the milliliters per hour to set the IV pump.

$$\frac{600 \text{ mg}}{60 \text{ min}} \left| \frac{200 \text{ (mL)}}{500 \text{ mg}} \right| \frac{60 \text{ min}}{1 \text{ (hr)}} \left| \frac{600 \times 2}{5 \times 1} \right| \frac{1200}{5} = 240 \frac{\text{mL}}{\text{hr}}$$

22. Random method:

$$\frac{2 \text{ mcg}}{\text{kg/min}} \left| \frac{250 \text{ (mL)}}{200 \text{ mg}} \right| \frac{1 \text{ mg}}{1000 \text{ mcg}} \left| \frac{60 \text{ min}}{1 \text{ (hr)}} \right| \frac{1 \text{ kg}}{2.2 \text{ lb}} \left| \frac{175 \text{ lb}}{} \right| = \frac{\text{mL}}{\text{hr}}$$

$$\frac{2 \times 25 \times 1 \times 6 \times 175}{20 \times 100 \times 2.2} \left| \frac{52500}{4400} \right| = 11.9 \text{ or } 12 \frac{\text{mL}}{\text{hr}}$$

23. Sequential method:

$$\frac{150 \text{ units}}{\text{kg/(day)}} \left| \frac{\text{(mL)}}{10,000 \text{ units}} \right| \frac{80 \text{ kg}}{} \left| \frac{15 \times 8}{100} \right| \frac{120}{100} = 1.2 \frac{\text{mL}}{\text{day}}$$

24. Random method:
Calculate the milliliters per hour to set the IV pump for the one minute administration.

$$\frac{500 \text{ mcg}}{\text{kg/min}} \left| \frac{250 \text{ (mL)}}{2.5 \text{ g}} \right| \frac{1 \text{ g}}{1000 \text{ mg}} \left| \frac{1 \text{ mg}}{1000 \text{ mcg}} \right| \frac{90 \text{ kg}}{} \left| \frac{60 \text{ min}}{1 \text{ (hr)}} \right| = \frac{\text{mL}}{\text{hr}}$$

$$\frac{5 \times 25 \times 1 \times 9 \times 6}{2.5 \times 10 \times 1} \left| \frac{6750}{25} \right| = 270 \frac{\text{mL}}{\text{hr}}$$

Calculate the milliliters per hour to set the IV pump for the four minute administration.

$$\frac{50 \text{ mcg}}{\text{kg/min}} \left| \frac{250 \text{ (mL)}}{2.5 \text{ g}} \right| \frac{1 \text{ g}}{1000 \text{ mg}} \left| \frac{1 \text{ mg}}{1000 \text{ mcg}} \right| \frac{90 \text{ kg}}{} \left| \frac{60 \text{ min}}{1 \text{ (hr)}} \right| = \frac{\text{mL}}{\text{hr}}$$

$$\frac{5 \times 25 \times 1 \times 9 \times 6}{2.5 \times 10 \times 10} \left| \frac{6750}{250} \right| = 27 \frac{\text{mL}}{\text{hr}}$$

25. Sequential method:

$$\frac{0.1 \text{ mg}}{\text{kg/(day)}} \left| \frac{5 \text{ (mL)}}{5 \text{ mg}} \right| \frac{35 \text{ kg}}{} \left| \frac{0.1 \times 35}{} \right| = 3.5 \frac{\text{mL}}{\text{day}}$$

Comprehensive Practice Problems

1. Sequential method:

$$\frac{0.125 \text{ mg} \mid \text{tablet}}{\mid 0.25 \text{ mg}} \frac{\mid 0.125}{\mid 0.25} = 0.5 \text{ tablet}$$

2. Random method:

$$\frac{0.5 \text{ g} \mid \text{tablet} \mid 1000 \text{ mg}}{\mid 500 \text{ mg} \mid 1 \text{ g}} \frac{\mid 0.5 \times 10 \mid 5}{\mid 5 \times 1 \mid 5} = 1 \text{ tablet}$$

3. Random method:

$$\frac{\frac{1}{150} \text{ gr} \mid \text{mL} \mid 60 \text{ mg}}{\mid 0.4 \text{ mg} \mid 1 \text{ gr}} \frac{\mid \frac{1}{150} \times \frac{60}{1} \mid \frac{60}{150} \mid 0.4}{\mid 0.4 \times 1 \mid 0.4 \mid 0.4} = 1 \text{ mL}$$

4. Sequential method:

$$\frac{500,000 \text{ units} \mid \text{mL} \mid 1 \text{ tsp}}{\mid 100,000 \text{ units} \mid 5 \text{ mL}} \frac{\mid 5 \times 1 \mid 5}{\mid 1 \times 5 \mid 5} = 1 \text{ tsp}$$

5. Sequential method:

$$\frac{50 \text{ mg} \mid \text{mL}}{\mid 100 \text{ mg}} \frac{\mid 5}{\mid 10} = 0.5 \text{ mL}$$

6. Sequential method:

$$\frac{2 \text{ mg} \mid 10 \text{ mL} \mid 75 \text{ kg}}{\text{kg} \mid 500 \text{ mg} \mid} \frac{\mid 2 \times 1 \times 75 \mid 150}{\mid 50 \mid 50} = 3 \text{ mL}$$

7. Sequential method:

$$\frac{2 \text{ mg} \mid 5 \text{ mL} \mid 1 \text{ kg} \mid 100 \text{ lb}}{\text{kg} \mid 500 \text{ mg} \mid 2.2 \text{ lb} \mid} \frac{\mid 2 \times 5 \times 1 \times 1 \mid 10}{\mid 5 \times 2.2 \mid 11} = 0.9 \text{ mL}$$

8. Sequential method:

$$\frac{1000 \text{ mL} \mid 15 \text{ gtt} \mid 1 \text{ hr}}{12 \text{ hr} \mid \text{mL} \mid 60 \text{ min}} \frac{\mid 100 \times 15 \times 1 \mid 1500}{\mid 12 \times 6 \mid 72} = \frac{20.8 \text{ or } 21 \text{ gtt}}{\text{min}}$$

9. Sequential method:

$$\frac{500 \text{ mL} \mid 15 \text{ gtt} \mid \text{min} \mid 1 \text{ hr}}{\mid \text{mL} \mid 21 \text{ gtt} \mid 60 \text{ min}} \frac{\mid 50 \times 15 \times 1 \mid 750}{\mid 21 \times 6 \mid 126} = 5.9 \text{ hr}$$

10. Sequential method:

$$\frac{1500 \text{ units} \mid 250 \text{ mL}}{\text{hr} \mid 25,000 \text{ units}} \frac{\mid 15 \times 25 \mid 375}{\mid 25 \mid 25} = \frac{15 \text{ mL}}{\text{hr}}$$

11. Sequential method:

$$\frac{1000 \text{ mL} \mid 15 \text{ gtt} \mid \text{min} \mid 1 \text{ hr}}{\mid \text{mL} \mid 50 \text{ gtt} \mid 60 \text{ min}} \frac{\mid 10 \times 15 \times 1 \mid 150}{\mid 5 \times 6 \mid 30} = 5 \text{ hr}$$

12. Sequential method:

$$\frac{8 \text{ units} \mid 250 \text{ mL}}{\text{hr} \mid 100 \text{ units}} \frac{\mid 8 \times 25 \mid 200}{\mid 10 \mid 10} = \frac{20 \text{ mL}}{\text{hr}}$$

13. Sequential method:

$$\frac{500 \text{ mL} \mid 10 \text{ gtt} \mid 1 \text{ hr}}{8 \text{ hr} \mid \text{mL} \mid 60 \text{ min}} \frac{\mid 50 \times 10 \times 1 \mid 500}{\mid 8 \times 6 \mid 48} = \frac{10.4 \text{ or } 10 \text{ gtt}}{\text{min}}$$

14. Random method:

$$\frac{2 \text{ mEq} \mid 10 \text{ mL} \mid 500 \text{ mL}}{100 \text{ mL} \mid 20 \text{ mEq} \mid} \frac{\mid 2 \times 1 \times 5 \mid 10}{\mid 1 \times 2 \mid 2} = 5 \text{ mL}$$

15. Random method:

$$\frac{44 \text{ mg}}{\text{hr}} \left| \frac{250 \text{ mL}}{1 \text{ g}} \right| \frac{1 \text{ g}}{1000 \text{ mg}} \left| \frac{44 \times 25 \times 1}{1 \times 100} \right| \frac{1100}{100} = \frac{11 \text{ mL}}{\text{hr}}$$

16. Sequential method:

$$\frac{140 \text{ mL}}{\text{hr}} \left| \frac{30 \text{ mg}}{1000 \text{ mL}} \right| \frac{14 \times 3}{10} \left| \frac{42}{10} \right. = \frac{4.2 \text{ mg}}{\text{hr}}$$

17. How many milliliters will you draw from the vial after reconstitution?
Sequential method:

$$\frac{750 \text{ mg}}{} \left| \frac{\text{mL}}{500 \text{ mg}} \right| \frac{75}{50} = 1.5 \text{ mL}$$

Calculate the milliliters per hour to set the IV pump.
Sequential method:

$$\frac{101.5 \text{ mL}}{30 \text{ min}} \left| \frac{60 \text{ min}}{1 \text{ hr}} \right| \frac{101.5 \times 6}{3 \times 1} \left| \frac{609}{3} \right. = \frac{203 \text{ mL}}{\text{hr}}$$

Calculate the drops per minute with a drop factor of 10 gtt/mL.
Sequential method:

$$\frac{203 \text{ mL}}{\text{hr}} \left| \frac{10 \text{ gtt}}{\text{mL}} \right| \frac{1 \text{ hr}}{60 \text{ min}} \left| \frac{203 \times 1 \times 1}{6} \right| \frac{203}{6} = \frac{33.83 \text{ or } 34 \text{ gtt}}{\text{min}}$$

18. How many milliliters will you draw from the vial after reconstitution?
Sequential method:

$$\frac{1.5 \text{ g}}{} \left| \frac{5 \text{ mL}}{3 \text{ g}} \right| \frac{1.5 \times 5}{3} \left| \frac{7.5}{3} \right. = 2.5 \text{ mL}$$

Calculate the milliliters per hour to set the IV pump.
Sequential method:

$$\frac{52.5 \text{ mL}}{20 \text{ min}} \left| \frac{60 \text{ min}}{1 \text{ hr}} \right| \frac{52.5 \times 6}{2 \times 1} \left| \frac{315}{2} \right. = \frac{157.5 \text{ or } 158 \text{ mL}}{\text{hr}}$$

Calculate the drops per minute with a drop factor of 20 gtt/mL.
Sequential method:

$$\frac{158 \text{ mL}}{\text{hr}} \left| \frac{20 \text{ gtt}}{\text{mL}} \right| \frac{1 \text{ hr}}{60 \text{ min}} \left| \frac{158 \times 2 \times 1}{6} \right| \frac{316}{6} = \frac{52.66 \text{ or } 53 \text{ gtt}}{\text{min}}$$

19. Random method:

$$\frac{4 \text{ mcg}}{\text{kg/min}} \left| \frac{250 \text{ mL}}{400 \text{ mg}} \right| \frac{1 \text{ mg}}{1000 \text{ mcg}} \left| \frac{60 \text{ min}}{1 \text{ hr}} \right| \frac{1 \text{ kg}}{2.2 \text{ lb}} \left| \frac{120 \text{ lb}}{} \right. = \frac{\text{mL}}{\text{hr}}$$

$$\frac{4 \times 25 \times 1 \times 6 \times 1 \times 12}{40 \times 10 \times 1 \times 2.2} \left| \frac{7200}{880} \right. = \frac{8.1 \text{ or } 8 \text{ mL}}{\text{hr}}$$

20. Random method:

$$\frac{0.8 \text{ mcg}}{\text{kg/min}} \left| \frac{500 \text{ mL}}{50 \text{ mg}} \right| \frac{1 \text{ mg}}{1000 \text{ mcg}} \left| \frac{1 \text{ kg}}{2.2 \text{ lb}} \right| \frac{143 \text{ lb}}{} \left| \frac{60 \text{ min}}{1 \text{ hr}} \right. = \frac{\text{mL}}{\text{hr}}$$

$$\frac{0.8 \times 5 \times 1 \times 1 \times 143 \times 6}{5 \times 10 \times 2.2 \times 1} \left| \frac{3432}{110} \right. = \frac{31.2 \text{ or } 31 \text{ mL}}{\text{hr}}$$

21. Sequential method:

$$\frac{500 \text{ mg}}{} \left| \frac{5 \text{ mL}}{250 \text{ mg}} \right| \frac{50 \times 5}{25} \left| \frac{250}{25} \right. = 10 \text{ mL}$$

22. Sequential method:

$$\frac{50 \text{ mg} \quad | \quad \text{tablets} \quad | \quad 5}{| \quad 100 \text{ mg} \quad | \quad 10} = 0.5 \text{ tablet}$$

23. Sequential method:

$$\frac{150 \text{ mg} \quad | \quad 100 \text{ mL} \quad | \quad 60 \text{ min} \quad | \quad 100 \times 6 \quad | \quad 600}{10 \text{ min} \quad | \quad 150 \text{ mg} \quad | \quad 1 \text{ hr} \quad | \quad 1 \times 1 \quad | \quad 1} = \frac{600 \text{ mL}}{\text{hr}}$$

24. Sequential method:

$$\frac{30 \text{ mg} \quad | \quad 5 \text{ mL} \quad | \quad 15 \text{ kg} \quad | \quad 3 \times 5 \times 15 \quad | \quad 225}{\text{kg} \quad | \quad 100 \text{ mg} \quad | \quad \quad | \quad 10 \quad | \quad 10} = 22.5 \text{ or } 23 \text{ mL}$$

25. Sequential method:
How many milligrams per day is the child receiving?

$$\frac{45 \text{ mg} \quad | \quad 35 \text{ kg} \quad | \quad 45 \times 35 \quad | \quad 1575}{\text{kg/day} \quad | \quad \quad | \quad \quad | \quad} = \frac{1575 \text{ mg}}{\text{day}}$$

How many milligrams per dose is the child receiving?

$$\frac{1575 \text{ mg} \quad | \quad \text{day} \quad | \quad 1575 \quad | \quad 787.5}{\text{day} \quad | \quad 2 \text{ doses} \quad | \quad 2 \quad |} = \frac{787.5 \text{ or } 788 \text{ mg}}{\text{dose}}$$

How many milliliters per dose will you give?

$$\frac{788 \text{ mg} \quad | \quad 5 \text{ mL} \quad | \quad 788 \times 5 \quad | \quad 3940}{\text{dose} \quad | \quad 400 \text{ mg} \quad | \quad 400 \quad | \quad 400} = \frac{9.85 \text{ or } 10 \text{ mL}}{\text{dose}}$$

Case Studies

This section contains case studies simulating typical orders that might be written for patients with selected disorders. In each case, the orders include multiple situations that require the nurse to perform clinical calculations before being able to implement the order. After reading the short scenario, read through the list of orders.

   Place a check mark in the box next to the physician's order that probably requires further calculations before implementing.

■ CASE STUDY 1 Congestive Heart Failure

A patient is admitted to the hospital with a diagnosis of dyspnea, peripheral edema with a 10-lb weight gain, and a history of congestive heart failure. The orders from the physician include:

- ❏ Bed rest in Fowler's position
- ❏ O_2 at 4 L/min per nasal cannula
- ❏ Chest x-ray, complete blood count, electrolyte panel, BUN, serum creatinine levels, and a digoxin level
- ❏ IV of D5W/$\frac{1}{2}$ NS at 50 mL/hr
- ❏ Daily AM weight
- ❏ Antiembolism stockings
- ❏ Furosemide 40 mg IV daily
- ❏ Digoxin 0.125 mg PO daily
- ❏ KCl 20 mEq PO tid
- ❏ Low-Na diet
- ❏ Restrict PO fluids to 1500 mL/day
- ❏ Vitals every 4h
- ❏ Accurate intake/output

Identify the orders that require calculations.

Set up and solve each problem using dimensional analysis.

1. Calculate gtt/min using microtubing (60 gtt/mL).

2. Calculate the weight gain in kilograms.

3. Calculate how many mL of Lasix the patient will receive IV from a multi-dose vial labeled 10 mg/mL.

4. Calculate how many tablets of digoxin the patient will receive from a unit dose of 0.25 mg/tablet.

5. Calculate how many tablets of K-Dur the patient will receive from a unit dose of 10 mEq/tablet.

■ CASE STUDY 2   COPD/Emphysema

A patient is admitted to the hospital with dyspnea and COPD exacerbation. The orders from the physician include:

❏ Stat ABGs, chest x-ray, complete blood count, and electrolytes
❏ IV D5W/$\frac{1}{2}$ NS 1000 mL/8 hr
❏ Aminophylline IV loading dose of 5.6 mg/kg over 30 minutes followed by 0.5 mg/kg/hr continuous IV
❏ O$_2$ at 2 L/min per nasal cannula
❏ Albuterol respiratory treatments every 4h
❏ Chest physiotherapy every 4h
❏ Erythromycin 800 mg IV every 6h
❏ Bed rest
❏ Accurate intake/output
❏ High-calorie, protein-rich diet in six small meals daily
❏ Encourage PO fluids to 3 L/day

Identify the orders that require calculations.

Set up and solve each problem using dimensional analysis.

1. Calculate mL/hr to set the IV pump.

2. Calculate mL/hr to set the IV pump for the loading dose of aminophylline for a patient weighing 140 lb. Aminophylline supply: 100 mg/100 mL D5W.

3. Calculate mL/hr to set the IV pump for the continuous dose of aminophylline for a patient weighing 140 lb. Aminophylline supply: 1 g/250 mL D5W.

4. Calculate mL/hr to set the IV pump to infuse erythromycin 800 mg. Erythromycin supply: 1-g vial to be reconstituted with 20 mL sterile water and further diluted in 250 mL NS to infuse over 1 hr.

5. Calculate the PO fluids in mL/shift.

■ CASE STUDY 3   Small Cell Lung Cancer

A patient with small cell lung cancer is admitted to the hospital with fever and dehydration. The orders from the physician include:

- ❑ O_2 at 2 L/min per nasal cannula
- ❑ Chest x-ray; complete blood count; electrolytes; blood, urine, and sputum cultures; BUN and serum creatinine levels; type and cross for 2 units of PRBCs
- ❑ IV D5W/$\frac{1}{2}$ NS 1000 mL with 10 mEq KCl at 125 mL/hr
- ❑ 2 units of PRBCs if Hg is below 8
- ❑ 6 pack of platelets if under 20,000
- ❑ Neupogen 5 mcg/kg SQ daily
- ❑ Gentamicin 80 mg IV every 8h
- ❑ Decadron 8 mg IV daily
- ❑ Fortaz 1 g IV every 8h
- ❑ Accurate intake/output
- ❑ Encourage PO fluids
- ❑ Vitals every 4h (call for temperature above 102°F)

Identify the orders that require calculations.

Set up and solve each problem using dimensional analysis.

1. Calculate gtt/min using macrotubing (20 gtt/mL).

2. Calculate how many mcg of Neupogen will be given SQ to a patient weighing 160 lb.

3. Calculate mL/hr to set the IV pump to infuse gentamicin. The vial is labeled 40 mg/mL and is to be further diluted in 100 mL D5W to infuse over 1 hr.

4. Calculate how many mL of Decadron the patient will receive from a vial labeled dexamethasone 4 mg/mL.

5. Calculate mL/hr to set the IV pump to infuse Fortaz 1 g over 30 minutes. Supply: Fortaz 1 g/50 mL.

■ CASE STUDY 4 Acquired Immunodeficiency Syndrome (AIDS)

A patient who is HIV+ and a Jehovah's Witness is admitted to the hospital with anemia, fever of unknown origin, and wasting syndrome with dehydration. The orders from the physician include:

- ❏ O$_2$ at 4 L/min per nasal cannula
- ❏ IV D5W/$\frac{1}{2}$ NS at 150 mL/hr
- ❏ CD4 and CD8 T-cell subset counts; erythrocyte sedimentation rate; complete blood count; urine, sputum, and stool cultures; chest x-ray
- ❏ Acyclovir 350 mg IV every 8h
- ❏ Neupogen 300 mcg SQ daily
- ❏ Epogen 100 units/kg SQ three times a week
- ❏ Megace 40 mg PO tid
- ❏ Zidovudine 100 mg PO every 4h
- ❏ Vancomycin 800 mg IV every 6h
- ❏ Respiratory treatments with pentamidine
- ❏ High-calorie, protein-rich diet in six small meals daily
- ❏ Encourage PO fluids to 3 L/day
- ❏ Accurate intake/output
- ❏ Daily AM weight

Identify the orders that require calculations.

Set up and solve each problem using dimensional analysis.

1. Calculate gtt/min using macrotubing (20 gtt/mL).

2. Calculate mL/hr to set the IV pump to infuse acyclovir 350 mg. Supply: 500-mg vial to be reconstituted with 10 mL sterile water and further diluted in 100 mL D5W to infuse over 1 hr.

3. Calculate how many mL of Neupogen will be given SQ. The vial is labeled 300 mcg/mL.

4. Calculate how many mL of Epogen will be given SQ to the patient weighing 100 lb. The vial is labeled 4000 units/mL.

5. Calculate how many mL/hr to set the IV pump to infuse vancomycin 800 mg. Supply: 1-g vials to be reconstituted with 10 mL NS and further diluted in 100 mL D5W to infuse over 60 min.

■ CASE STUDY 5   Sickle Cell Anemia

A patient is admitted to the hospital in sickle cell crisis. The orders from the physician include:

- ❏ Bed rest with joint support
- ❏ O_2 at 2 L/min per nasal cannula
- ❏ Complete blood count, erythrocyte sedimentation rate, serum iron levels, and chest x-ray
- ❏ IV D5W/$\frac{1}{2}$ NS at 150 mL/hr
- ❏ Zofran 8 mg IV every 8h
- ❏ Morphine sulfate 5 mg IV prn
- ❏ Hydrea 10 mg/kg/day PO
- ❏ Folic acid 0.5 mg daily PO
- ❏ Encourage 3000 mL/daily PO

Identify the orders that require calculations.

Set up and solve each problem using dimensional analysis.

1. Calculate gtt/min using macrotubing (10 gtt/mL).

2. Calculate mL/hr to set the IV pump to infuse Zofran 8 mg. Supply: Zofran 8 mg in 50 mL D5W to infuse over 15 min.

3. Calculate how many mL of morphine sulfate will be given IV. The syringe is labeled 10 mg/mL.

4. Calculate how many mg/day of Hydrea will be given PO to the patient weighing 125 lb.

5. Calculate how many tablets of folic acid will be given PO. Supply: 1 mg/tablet.

■ CASE STUDY 6   Deep Vein Thrombosis

A patient is admitted to the hospital with right leg erythema and edema to R/O DVT. The orders from the physician include:

- ❏ Bed rest with right leg elevated
- ❏ Warm, moist heat to right leg with Aqua-K pad
- ❏ Doppler ultrasonography
- ❏ Partial thromboplastin time (PTT) and prothrombin time (PT)
- ❏ IV D5W/$\frac{1}{2}$ NS with 20 mEq KCl at 50 mL/hr
- ❏ Heparin 5000 units IV push followed by continuous IV infusion of 1000 units/hr
- ❏ Lasix 20 mg IV bid
- ❏ Morphine 5 mg IV every 4h

Identify the orders that require calculations.

Set up and solve each problem using dimensional analysis.

1. Calculate gtt/min using microtubing (60 gtt/mL).

2. Calculate how many mL of heparin the patient will receive IV from a multidose vial labeled 10,000 units/mL.

3. Calculate mL/hr to set the IV pump for the continuous dose of heparin. Heparin supply: 25,000 units/250 mL D5W.

4. Calculate how many mL of Lasix the patient will receive IV from a multidose vial labeled 10 mg/mL.

5. Calculate how many mL of morphine the patient will receive from a syringe labeled 10 mg/mL.

■ CASE STUDY 7   Bone Marrow Transplant

A patient is admitted to the hospital with a rash after an allogeneic bone marrow transplant. The orders from the physician include:

❏ IV D5W/$\frac{1}{2}$ NS with 20 mEq KCl/L at 80 mL/hr
❏ Complete blood count; electrolytes; sputum, urine, and stool cultures; blood cultures ×3; liver panel; BUN; and creatinine
❏ Vitals every 4h
❏ Strict intake/output
❏ Fortaz 2 g IV every 8h
❏ Vancomycin 1 g IV every 6h
❏ Claforan 1 g IV every 12h
❏ Erythromycin 800 mg IV every 6h

Identify the orders that require calculations.

Set up and solve each problem using dimensional analysis.

1. Calculate how many mEq/hr of KCl the patient will receive IV.

2. Calculate mL/hr to set the IV pump to infuse Fortaz 2 g. Supply: Fortaz 2-g vial to be reconstituted with 10 mL of sterile water and further diluted in 50 mL D5W to infuse over 30 min.

3. Calculate mL/hr to set the IV pump to infuse vancomycin 1 g. Supply: vancomycin 500-mg vial to be reconstituted with 10 mL of sterile water and further diluted in 100 mL of D5W to infuse over 60 min.

4. Calculate mL/hr to set the IV pump to infuse Claforan 1 g. Supply: Claforan 600 mg/4 mL to be further diluted with 100 mL D5W to infuse over 1 hr.

5. Calculate mL/hr to set the IV pump to infuse erythromycin 800 mg. Supply: Erythromycin 1-g vial to be diluted with 20 mL sterile water and further diluted in 250 mL of NS to infuse over 60 min.

■ CASE STUDY 8   Pneumonia

A patient is admitted to the hospital with fever, cough, chills, and dyspnea to rule out pneumonia. The orders from the physician include:

- ❏ IV 600 mL D5W every 8h
- ❏ Intake/output
- ❏ Vitals every 4h
- ❏ Complete blood count, electrolytes, chest x-ray, ABGs, sputum specimen, blood cultures, and bronchoscopy
- ❏ Bed rest
- ❏ Humidified O_2 at 4 L/min per nasal cannula
- ❏ High-calorie diet
- ❏ Encourage oral fluids of 2000 to 3000 mL/day
- ❏ Pulse oximetry every AM
- ❏ Clindamycin 400 mg IV every 6h
- ❏ Albuterol respiratory treatments
- ❏ Guaifenesin 200 mg PO every 4h
- ❏ Terbutaline 2.5 mg PO tid
- ❏ MS Contrin 30 mg PO every 4h prn

Identify the orders that require calculations.

Set up and solve each problem using dimensional analysis.

1. Calculate mL/hr to set the IV pump to infuse clindamycin 400 mg. Supply: Clindamycin 600 mg/4 mL to be further diluted with 50 mL D5W to infuse over 1 hr.

2. Calculate gtt/min to infuse the clindamycin using macrotubing (20 gtt/mL).

3. Calculate how many mL of guaifenesin the patient will receive from a stock bottle labeled 30 mg/tsp.

4. Calculate how many tablets of terbutaline the patient will receive from a unit dose of 5 mg/tablet.

5. Calculate how many tablets of MS Contrin the patient will receive from a unit dose of 30 mg/tablet.

■ CASE STUDY 9   Pain

A patient is admitted to the hospital with intractable bone pain secondary to prostate cancer. The orders from the physician include:

- ❏ IV D5W/$\frac{1}{2}$ NS with 20 mEq KCl/L at 60 mL/hr
- ❏ IV 500 mL NS with 25 mg Dilaudid and 50 mg Thorazine at 21 mL/hr
- ❏ Heparin 25,000 units/250 mL D5W at 11 mL/hr
- ❏ Bed rest
- ❏ Do not resuscitate
- ❏ O$_2$ at 2 L/min per nasal cannula
- ❏ Bumex 2 mg IV every AM after albumin infusion
- ❏ Albumin 12.5 g IV every AM

Identify the orders that require calculations.

Set up and solve each problem using dimensional analysis.

1. Calculate how many mEq/hr of KCl the patient is receiving.

2. Calculate how many mg/hr of Dilaudid the patient is receiving.

3. Calculate how many mg/hr of Thorazine the patient is receiving.

4. Calculate how many units/hr of heparin the patient is receiving.

5. Calculate how many mL of Bumex the patient will receive from a stock dose of 0.25 mg/mL.

■ CASE STUDY 10   Cirrhosis

A patient is admitted to the hospital with ascites, stomach pain, dyspnea, and a history of cirrhosis of the liver. The orders from the physician include:

- ❏ IV D5W/$\frac{1}{2}$ NS with 20 mEq KCl at 125 mL/hr
- ❏ IV Zantac 150 mg/250 mL NS at 11 mL/hr
- ❏ O$_2$ at 2 L/min per nasal cannula
- ❏ Type and crossmatch for 2 units of packed red blood cells, complete blood count, liver panel, PT/PTT, SMA-12.
- ❏ Carafate 1 g every 4h PO
- ❏ Vitamin K 10 mg SQ every AM
- ❏ Spironolactone 50 mg PO bid
- ❏ Lasix 80 mg IV every AM
- ❏ Measure abdominal girth every AM
- ❏ Sodium restriction to 500 mg/day
- ❏ Fluid restriction to 1500 mL/day

Identify the orders that require calculations.

Set up and solve each problem using dimensional analysis.

1. Calculate the gtt/min using macrotubing (20 gtt/mL).

2. Calculate the mg/hr of Zantac the patient is receiving.

3. Calculate how many mL of vitamin K the patient will receive SQ from a unit dose labeled 10 mg/mL.

4. Calculate how many tablets of spironolactone the patient will receive from a unit dose labeled 25 mg/tablet.

5. Calculate how many mL of Lasix the patient will receive from a unit dose labeled 10 mg/mL.

■ CASE STUDY 11   **Hyperemesis Gravidarum**

A 14-year-old patient is admitted to the hospital with weight loss and dehydration secondary to hyperemesis gravidarum. The orders from the physician include:

- ❏ Bed rest with bathroom privileges
- ❏ Obtain weight daily
- ❏ Vital every 4h
- ❏ Test urine for ketones
- ❏ Urinalysis, complete blood count, electrolytes, liver enzymes, and bilirubin
- ❏ NPO for 48 hr, then advance diet to clear liquid, full liquid, and as tolerated
- ❏ IV D5 $\frac{1}{2}$ NS at 150 mL/hr for 8 hr, then decrease to 100 mL/hr
- ❏ Observe for signs of metabolic acidosis, jaundice, or hemorrhage
- ❏ Monitor intake and output
- ❏ Droperidol (Inapsine) 1 mg IV every 4h prn for nausea
- ❏ Metoclopramide (Reglan) 20 mg IV in 50 mL of D5W to infuse over 15 min
- ❏ Diphenhydramine (Benadryl) 25 mg IV every 3h prn for nausea
- ❏ Dexamethasone (Decadron) 4 mg IV every 6h

Identify the orders that require calculations.

Set up and solve each problem using dimensional analysis.

1. Calculate gtt/min using macrotubing (20 gtt/mL) to infuse 150 mL/hr, then 100 mL/hr.

2. Calculate how many mL of droperidol the patient will receive IV. Supply: 2.5 mg/mL

3. Calculate mL/hr to set the IV pump to infuse metoclopramide (Reglan) 20 mg in 50 mL of D5W to infuse over 15 min.

4. Calculate how many mL of diphenhydramine (Benadryl) the patient will receive IV. Supply: 10 mg/mL.

5. Calculate how many mL of dexamethasone (Decadron) the patient will receive IV. Supply: 4 mg/mL.

■ **CASE STUDY 12**   **Preeclampsia**

A nulliparous female is admitted to the hospital with pregnancy-induced hypertension. The orders from the physician include:

❏ Complete bed rest in left lateral position
❏ Insert Foley catheter and check hourly for protein and specific gravity
❏ Daily weight
❏ Methyldopa (Aldomet) 250 mg PO tid
❏ Hydralazine (Apresoline) 5 mg IV every 20 min for blood pressure over 160/100
❏ Complete blood count, liver enzymes, chemistry panel, clotting studies, type and crossmatch, and urinalysis
❏ Magnesium sulfate 4 g in 250 mL D5LR loading dose to infuse over 30 min
❏ Magnesium sulfate 40 g in 1000 mL LR to infuse at 1 g/hr
❏ Keep calcium gluconate and intubation equipment at the bedside
❏ Nifedipine (Procardia) 10 mg sublingual for blood pressure over 160/100 and repeat in 15 min if needed.
❏ Keep lights dimmed and maintain a quiet environment
❏ Monitor blood pressure, pulse, and respiratory rate, fetal heart rate (FHR) contractions every 15 to 30 min, and deep tendon reflexes (DTR) hourly
❏ Monitor intake and output, proteinuria, presence of headache, visual disturbances, and epigastric pain hourly
❏ Restrict hourly fluid intake to 100 to 125 mL/hr

Identify the orders that require calculations.

Set up and solve each problem using dimensional analysis.

1. Calculate how many tablets of methyldopa (Aldomet) will be given PO. Supply: 500 mg/tablet.

2. Calculate how many mL of hydralazine (Apresoline) will be given IV. Supply: 20 mg/mL.

3. Calculate mL/hr to set the IV pump to infuse magnesium sulfate 4 g in 250 mL D5W loading dose to infuse over 30 min.

4. Calculate mL/hr to set the IV pump to infuse magnesium sulfate 40 g in 1000 mL LR to infuse at 1 g/hr.

5. Calculate how many capsules of nifedipine (Procardia) will be needed to give the sublingual dose. Supply: 10 mg/capsule.

■ CASE STUDY 13   Premature Labor

A 35-year-old female in the 30th week of gestation is admitted to the hospital in premature labor. The orders from the physician include:

- ❏ Bed rest in left lateral position
- ❏ Monitor intake and output
- ❏ Daily weights
- ❏ Continuous fetal monitoring
- ❏ Monitor blood pressure, pulse rate, respirations, fetal heart rate, uterine contraction pattern, and neurologic reflexes
- ❏ Keep calcium gluconate at the bedside
- ❏ Initiate magnesium sulfate 4 g in 250 mL LR loading dose over 20 min, then 2 g in 250 mL LR at 2 g/hr until contractions stop
- ❏ Continue tocolytic therapy with terbutaline (Brethine) 0.25 mg SQ every 30 min for 2 hr after contractions stop
- ❏ Give nifedipine (Procardia) 10 mg sublingual now, then 20 mg PO every 6h after infusion of magnesium sulfate and contractions have stopped
- ❏ Betamethasone 12 mg IM × 2 doses 12 hr apart
- ❏ IV LR 1000 mL over 8 hr

Identify the orders that require calculations.

Set up and solve each problem using dimensional analysis.

1. Calculate mL/hr to set the IV pump to infuse the loading dose magnesium sulfate 4 g in 250 mL LR over 20 min and the 2 g/hr maintenance dose.

2. Calculate how many mL of terbutaline (Brethine) will be given SQ. Supply: 1 mg/mL.

3. Calculate how many capsules of nifedipine (Procardia) will be given PO every 6h. Supply: 10 mg/capsule.

4. Betamethasone 12 mg IM × 2 doses 12 hr apart. Supply: 6 mg/mL.

5. Calculate mL/hr to set the IV pump to infuse LR 1000 mL over 8 hr.

■ CASE STUDY 14   Cystic Fibrosis

A 10-year-old child weighing 65 lb is admitted to the hospital with pulmonary exacerbation. The orders from the physician include:

❏ Complete blood count with differential, ABGs, chest x-ray, urinalysis, chemistry panel, and sputum culture
❏ IV 0.9% normal saline at 75 mL/hr
❏ Daily weights
❏ Monitor vitals every 4h
❏ Oxygen at 2 L/min with pulse oximetry checks to maintain oxygen saturation above 92%
❏ Pancrease 2 capsules PO with meals and snacks
❏ High-calorie, high-protein diet
❏ Multivitamin 1 tablet PO daily
❏ Tagamet 30 mg/kg/day PO in four divided doses with meals and HS with a snack.
❏ Clindamycin 10 mg/kg IV every 6h
❏ Postural drainage and percussion after aerosolized treatments
❏ Albuterol treatments with 2 inhalations every 4h to 6h
❏ Terbutaline PO 2.5 mg every 6h
❏ Tobramycin 1.5 mg/kg every 6h
❏ Tobramycin peak and trough levels after fourth dose

Identify the orders that require calculations.

Set up and solve each problem using dimensional analysis.

1. Calculate gtt/min using macrotubing (15 gtt/mL).

2. Calculate how many tablets of Tagamet will be given PO with meals and HS snack. Supply: 200 mg/tablet.

3. Calculate how many mg of clindamycin the patient will receive, how many mL to draw from the vial, and mL/hr to set the IV pump. Supply: 150 mg/mL vial to be further diluted in 50 mL of NS and infused over 20 min.

4. Calculate how many tablets of terbutaline will be given PO. Supply: 2.5 mg/tablet.

5. Calculate how many mg of tobramycin the patient will receive, how many mL to draw from the vial, and mL/hr to set the IV pump. Supply: 40 mg/mL vial to be further diluted in 50 mL of NS and infused over 30 min.

■ CASE STUDY 15   Respiratory Syncytial Virus (RSV)

A 2-year-old child weighing 30 lb is admitted to the hospital for severe respiratory distress. The orders from the physician include:

- ❏ Complete blood count with differential, electrolytes, blood culture, chest x-ray, and nasal washing
- ❏ Humidified oxygen therapy to keep oxygen saturation >92%
- ❏ Continuous pulse oximetry
- ❏ IV D5W$\frac{1}{2}$NS at 50 mL/hr
- ❏ Elevate HOB
- ❏ Vitals every 2h
- ❏ Contact isolation
- ❏ Cardiorespiratory monitor
- ❏ Strict intake and output with urine specific gravities
- ❏ Acetaminophen elixir 120 mg every 4h prn for temperature above 101°F
- ❏ Aminophylline loading dose of 5 mg/kg to infuse over 30 min and maintenance dose of 0.8 mg/kg/hr
- ❏ Ribavirin (Virazole) inhalation therapy × 12 hr/day
- ❏ NPO with respiratory rate above 60
- ❏ RespiGam 750 mg/kg IV monthly
- ❏ Pediapred 1.5 mg/kg/day in three divided doses
- ❏ Ampicillin 100 mg/kg/day in divided doses every 6h

Identify the orders that require calculations.

Set up and solve each problem using dimensional analysis.

1. Calculate how many mL of acetaminophen elixir the patient will receive. Supply: 120 mg/5 mL.

2. Calculate how many mg of aminophylline the patient will receive and the mL/hr to set the IV pump for the loading dose, then calculate the mL/hr to set the IV pump for the maintenance dose. Supply: 250 mg/100 mL.

3. Calculate how many mg of RespiGam the patient will receive IV on a monthly infusion.

4. Calculate how many mL/dose of Pediapred the patient will receive. Supply: 15 mg/5 mL.

5. Calculate how many mg/dose of ampicillin the patient will receive IV, how many mL to draw from the vial, and mL/hr to set the IV pump. Supply: 1-g vials to be diluted with 10 mL of NS and further diluted in 50 mL NS to infuse over 30 min.

■ CASE STUDY 16   **Leukemia**

A 14-year-old child is admitted to the hospital with fever of unknown origin (FUO) after chemotherapy administration. The orders from the physician include:

❏ Complete blood count with differential, bone marrow aspiration, chemistry panel, PT/PTT, blood cultures, urinalysis, and type and crossmatch
❏ Regular diet as tolerated
❏ Vitals every 4h
❏ Daily weights
❏ Monitor intake and output
❏ Type and cross for 2 units PRBCs
❏ Irradiate all blood products
❏ Infuse 6 pack of platelets for counts under 20,000
❏ IV D5W/NS with 20 mEq KCl 1000 mL/8 hr
❏ Allopurinol 200 mg PO tid
❏ Fortaz 1 g IV every 6h
❏ Aztreonam (Azactam) 2 g IV every 12h
❏ Flagyl 500 mg IV every 8h
❏ Acetaminophen two tablets every 4h prn

Identify the orders that require calculations.

Set up and solve each problem using dimensional analysis.

1. Calculate mL/hr to set the IV pump.

2. Calculate how many tablets of allopurinol will be given PO.
   Supply: 100 mg/tablet.

3. Calculate how many mL/hr to set the IV pump to infuse Fortaz. Supply: 1-g vial to be diluted with 10 mL of sterile water and further diluted in 50 mL NS to infuse over 30 min.

4. Calculate how many mL of aztreonam to draw from the vial. Supply: 2-g vial to be diluted with 10 mL of sterile water and further diluted in 100 mL NS to infuse over 60 min.

5. Calculate how many mL/hr to set the IV pump to infuse Flagyl. Supply: 500 mg/100 mL to infuse over 1 hr.

■ CASE STUDY 17   Sepsis

A neonate born at 32 weeks' gestation (weight 2005 g) is admitted to the Neonatal Intensive Care Unit (NICU) with a diagnosis of sepsis. The orders from the physician include:

- ❏ Admit to NICU with continuous cardiorespiratory monitoring
- ❏ Complete blood counts, blood and urine cultures, chest x-ray, bilirubin, ABGs, theophylline levels, and lumbar puncture
- ❏ Strict intake and output
- ❏ Daily weight
- ❏ Vitals every 3h
- ❏ NG breast milk diluted with sterile water 120 mL/day with feedings every 3h
- ❏ IV D10 and 20% lipids 120 mL/kg/day
- ❏ Aminophylline 5 mg/kg IV every 6h
- ❏ Cefotaxime (Claforan) 50 mg/kg every 12h
- ❏ Vancomycin 10 mg/kg/dose every 12h

Identify the orders that require calculations.

Set up and solve each problem using dimensional analysis.

1. Calculate how many mL the child will receive with every feeding.

2. Calculate how many mL/hr the child will receive IV.

3. Calculate how many mg of aminophylline the child will receive every 6h. Calculate how many mL/hr you will set the IV pump. Supply: 50 mg/ 10 mL to infuse over 5 min.

4. Calculate how many mg of cefotaxime the child will receive every 12 hr. Calculate how many mL/hr you will set the IV pump. Supply: 40 mg/mL to infuse over 30 min.

5. Calculate how many mg of vancomycin the child will receive every 12 hr. Calculate how many mL/hr you will set the IV pump. Supply: 5 mg/mL to infuse over 1 hr.

■ CASE STUDY 18   Bronchopulmonary Dysplasia

A neonate born at 24 weeks' gestation diagnosed with respiratory distress syndrome and respiratory failure is now 28 weeks' gestation (weight 996 g) with bronchopulmonary dysplasia. This child remains in the Neonatal Intensive Care Unit (NICU) on oxygen therapy and enteral feedings. The orders from the physician include:

- ❑ Complete blood count, chemistry panel, ABGs, chest x-ray, CPPD with nebulizations, glucose monitoring, caffeine citrate levels, and newborn screen
- ❑ NG feedings with Special Care with Iron 120 kcal/kg/day
- ❑ Chlorothiazide (Diuril) 10 mg/kg/day PO
- ❑ Fer-In-Sol 2 mg/kg/day
- ❑ Vitamin E 25 units/kg/day in divided doses every 12h
- ❑ Caffeine citrate 5 mg/kg/dose daily

Identify the orders that require calculations.

Set up and solve each problem using dimensional analysis.

1. Calculate how many total calories the child will receive daily. Calculate how many mL/day the child will receive. Supply: 24 kcal/oz.

2. Calculate how many mg of chlorothiazide the child will receive daily. Calculate how many mL/day the child will receive. Supply: 250 mg/5 mL.

3. Calculate how many mg of Fer-In-Sol the child will receive daily. Calculate how many mL/day the child will receive. Supply: 15 mg/0.6 mL.

4. Calculate how many units/dose of vitamin E the child will receive every 12 hr. Calculate how many mL/dose the child will receive. Supply: 67 units/mL.

5. Calculate how many mg of caffeine citrate the child will receive daily. Calculate how many mL/dose the child will receive. Supply: 10 mg/mL.

■ CASE STUDY 19   **Cerebral Palsy**

A 13-year-old child (weight 38 kg) with cerebral palsy being cared for in a children's facility is admitted to the hospital for seizure evaluation. The orders from the physician include:

- ❏ Complete blood count, chemistry panel, urinalysis, dilantin levels, EEG, and CT scan
- ❏ Vitals every 4h
- ❏ Seizure precautions
- ❏ Lactulose 3 g PO tid
- ❏ Valproic acid (Depakote) 30 mg/kg/day PO in three divided doses
- ❏ Diazepam (Valium) 2.5 mg PO daily
- ❏ Chlorothiazide (Thiazide) 250 mg PO daily
- ❏ Phenytoin (Dilantin) 5 mg/kg/day PO in three divided doses

Identify the orders that require calculations.

Set up and solve each problem using dimensional analysis.

1. Calculate how many mL of lactulose the child will receive. Supply: 10 g/15 mL.

2. Calculate how many tablets of Depakote the child will receive per dose. Supply: 125 mg/tablet.

3. Calculate how many tablets of diazepam the child will receive per dose. Supply: 5 mg/tablet.

4. Calculate how many tablets of chlorothiazide the child will receive per dose. Supply: 250 mg/tablet.

5. Calculate how many mL of Dilantin the child will receive per dose. Supply: 125 mg/5 mL.

■ CASE STUDY 20   **Hyperbilirubinemia**

A 4-day-old neonate born at 35 weeks' gestation (weight 2210 g) is readmitted to the hospital for treatment of dehydration and jaundice with a bilirubin level of 21 mg/dL. The orders from the physician include:

- ❏ Phototherapy and exchange transfusion through an umbilical venous catheter
- ❏ Total and indirect bilirubin levels, electrolytes, complete blood count, and type and crossmatch
- ❏ Continuous cardiorespiratory monitoring
- ❏ Vitals every 2h
- ❏ Monitor intake and output

❑ Albumin 5% infusion 1 g/kg 1 hr before exchange
❑ Ampicillin 100 mg/kg/dose IV every 12h
❑ Gentamicin 4 mg/kg/dose IV every 12h
❑ NPO before exchange, then 120 mL/kg/day formula
❑ IV D10W 120 mL/kg/day

Identify the orders that require calculations.

Set up and solve each problem using dimensional analysis.

1. Calculate how many g of albumin the infant will receive before exchange therapy.

2. Calculate how many mg/dose of ampicillin the infant will receive every 12 hr. Calculate how many mL the infant will receive. Supply: 250 mg/5 mL IV push over 5 min.

3. Calculate how many mg/dose of gentamicin the infant will receive every 12 hr. Calculate how many mL the infant will receive. Supply: 2 mg/mL.

4. Calculate how many mL/day of formula the infant will receive.

5. Calculate how many mL/hr to set the IV pump.

■ CASE STUDY 21   **Spontaneous Abortion**

A 31-year-old female is admitted to the hospital to control severe hemorrhage after a spontaneous abortion. The orders from the physician include:

❑ CBC to determine blood loss
❑ WBC with differential to rule out infection
❑ Type and crossmatch for 2 units of blood
❑ Obtain Coombs' test to determine Rh status
❑ Administer Rhogam 300 mcg IM if patient is Rh-negative with a negative indirect Coombs' test
❑ IV D5/0.9% NS at 100 mL/hr
❑ IV oxytocin (Pitocin) 10 Units infused at 20 mU/min
❑ Prepare for a dilatation and curettage (D&C)
❑ Complete bed rest. Monitor bedpan for contents for intrauterine material
❑ Administer meperidine (Demerol) 50 mg IM every 4h for severe discomfort
❑ Administer ibuprofen 400 mg PO every 6h for mild discomfort
❑ Monitor vital signs every 4h for 24 hr
❑ Monitor urine output
❑ Note the amount, color, and odor of vaginal bleeding

Identify the orders that require calculations.

Set up and solve each problem using dimensional analysis.

1. Calculate how many mL of Rhogam the patient will receive.
   Supply: Rhogam 300 mcg/mL vial. Administer into the deltoid muscle within 72 hr of abortion.

2. Calculate gtt/min using macrotubing (15 gtt/mL).

3. Calculate how many mL/hr to set the IV pump to infuse oxytocin 10 units. Supply: Oxytocin 10 units in 500 mL D5/NS.

4. Calculate how many mL of meperidine (Demerol) will be given IM. The prefilled syringe is labeled 100 mg/mL.

5. Calculate how many tablets of ibuprofen will be given PO.
   Supply: 200 mg/tablet.

■ CASE STUDY 22   **Bipolar Disorder**

A 25-year-old female is brought to the hospital by her friends after she fainted at the PowerShop. Her friends reported that she has been very sad, withdrawn, and not involved in any of her usual activities for some time but had suddenly become "full of energy" at the PowerShop. The orders from the physician include:

❑ CBC and electrolytes
❑ WBC with differential
❑ BUN and creatinine
❑ Liver panel
❑ Lithium levels
❑ IV 0.9% NS at 75 mL/hr
❑ Lithium 300 mg PO tid
❑ Clonazepam 0.5 mg PO bid; increase to 1 mg PO bid after 3 days
❑ Doxepin 50 mg PO tid
❑ Intake and output

Identify the orders that require calculations.

Set up and solve each problem using dimensional analysis.

1. Calculate the gtt/min using macrotubing (20 gtt/mL).

2. Calculate how many capsules of lithium will be given PO. Supply: 150 mg/capsule.

3. Calculate how many tablets of clonazepam will be given PO.
   Supply: 0.5-mg tablets.

4. Calculate how many tablets of clonazepam will be given PO after 3 days.
   Supply: 0.5-mg tablets.

5. Calculate how many tablets of doxepin will be given PO. Supply:
   25-mg tablets.

■ CASE STUDY 23   Anorexia Nervosa

A 17-year-old female high school student is admitted by her parents for self-induced starvation, vomiting, and laxative abuse. The 12-week hospital stay is for management of diet with a 1- to 2-lb/week weight gain goal. The orders from the physician include:

❑ DSM-IV evaluation
❑ Nutritional consult for 1500-calorie diet advance to 3500 calories over
   12 weeks
❑ CBC, platelet count, and sedimentation rate
❑ WBC with differential
❑ Electrolytes, BUN, and creatinine
❑ Liver enzymes
❑ Urinalysis
❑ ECG
❑ Daily weight
❑ Intake and output
❑ 1000 mL IV D5/LR with 20 mEq K+ to infuse over 8 hr
❑ Olanzapine (Zyprexa) 10 mg PO HS
❑ Fluoxetine (Prozac) 60 mg/day PO every AM
❑ Amitriptyline 25 mg PO qid
❑ Cyproheptadine 32 mg/day PO in 4 divided doses

Identify the orders that require calculations.

Set up and solve each problem using dimensional analysis.

1. Calculate how many mL/hr to set the IV pump.

2. Calculate how many tablets of olanzapine (Zyprexa) will be given at HS.
   Supply: 5-mg tablets.

3. Calculate how many mL of fluoxetine (Prozac) will be given PO.
   Supply: 20 mg/5 mL.

4. Calculate how many tablets of amitriptyline will be given PO. Supply: 10 mg/5 mL.

5. Calculate how many mL of cyproheptadine will be given PO. Supply: 2 mg/5 mL.

■ CASE STUDY 24   Clinical Depression

A 44-year-old successful businessman with a wife and two children, and diagnosed with clinical depression, has received several months of treatment with antidepressants and psychotherapy. The depression has not responded to therapy. He has become suicidal, and he has agreed to try electroconvulsive therapy (also called ECT). The orders from the physician include:

- ❏ Admit for ECT
- ❏ CBC and urinalysis
- ❏ ECG
- ❏ NPO after midnight
- ❏ Obtain AM weight
- ❏ Obtain baseline vitals 60 min before procedure
- ❏ Start IV D5/0.45% at 100 mL/hr
- ❏ Administer glycopyrrolate (Robinul) 4.4 mcg/kg IM 30 min preoperatively
- ❏ Zoloft 50 mg PO every AM
- ❏ Sinequan 25 mg PO tid
- ❏ Parnate 30 mg/day PO in 2 divided doses

Identify the orders that require calculations.

Set up and solve each problem using dimensional analysis.

1. Calculate the gtt/min using macrotubing (10 gtt/mL).

2. Calculate how many mL of glycopyrrolate (Robinul) will be given IM. Supply: 200 mcg/mL. Patient weight: 175 lb.

3. Calculate how many tablets of sertraline (Zoloft) will be given PO. Supply: 50-mg tablets.

4. Calculate how many capsules of doxepin (Sinequan) will be given PO. Supply: 25-mg capsules.

5. Calculate how many tablets of tranylcypromine (Parnate) will be given PO. Supply: 10-mg tablets.

■ CASE STUDY 25   Alzheimer's Disease

A 62-year-old executive is experiencing difficulty remembering and perform-
ing familiar tasks, problems with abstract thinking, and changes in mood and
behavior. He is hospitalized for evaluation. The orders from the physician
include:

❏ CT of the brain
❏ EEG and cerebral blood flow studies
❏ CBC and electrolytes
❏ Cerebrospinal fluid analysis
❏ Urinalysis
❏ 1000 mL IV D5/0.45% NS to infuse over 8 hr
❏ Donepezil (Aricept) 5 mg PO HS
❏ Thioridazine (Mellaril) 25 mg PO tid
❏ Imipramine (Tofranil) 50 mg PO qid
❏ Temazepam (Restoril) 7.5 mg PO HS

Identify the orders that require calculations.

Set up and solve each problem using dimensional analysis.

1. Calculate gtt/min using macrotubing (15 gtt/mL).

2. Calculate how many tablets of donepezil (Aricept) will be given PO.
   Supply: 5-mg tablets.

3. Calculate how many tablets of thioridazine (Mellaril) will be given PO.
   Supply: 25-mg tablets.

4. Calculate how many tablets of imipramine (Tofranil) will be given PO.
   Supply: 25-mg tablets.

5. Calculate how many tablets of temazepam (Restoril) will be given PO.
   Supply: 15-mg tablets.

■ CASE STUDY 26   Otitis Media

An 18-month-old child is seen in the nurse practitioner's office for reoccurring otitis media and fever. The child's weight is 23 lb. The orders from the nurse practitioner include:

❑ Amoxicillin 45 mg/kg/day PO in divided doses every 12 h
❑ Acetaminophen (Tylenol) 120 mg PO every 4 h alternating with Ibuprofen 5 mg/kg PO every 6 h if temperature is 102.5° F or below and 10 mg/kg if temperature is greater than 102.5° F
❑ Cetirizine (Zyrtec) 2.5 mg PO every 12 h
❑ Pedialyte 75 mL per kg PO not to exceed more than 100 mL in any 20-minute period during the first 8 hr

Identify the orders that require calculations.

Set up and solve each problem using dimensional analysis.

1. Calculate how many mL/dose of amoxicillin will be given PO. Supply: amoxicillin 125 mg/5 mL solution.

2. Calculate how many mL of acetaminophen (Tylenol) will be given PO for a temperature of 102°. Supply: acetaminophen 100 mg/mL solution.

3. Calculate how many mL of ibuprofen will be given PO for a temperature of 102°. Supply: ibuprofen 100 mg/5 mL solution.

4. Calculate how many mL of Zyrtec will be given PO. Supply: Zyrtec 1 mg/mL.

5. Calculate how many mL/hr/8 hr of Pedialyte the patient will receive PO during the first 8 h.

■ CASE STUDY 27   Seizures

An 8-year-old child is admitted to the pediatric hospital with seizures secondary to a head injury following a fall on the playground. The child's weight is 60 lb. The orders from the physician include:

❑ Admit to pediatric intensive care
❑ Bedrest in quiet, darken environment
❑ Complete blood count, chemistry panel, urinalysis, EEG, skull and neck x-ray and CT scan
❑ Vitals every 2h
❑ Monitor intake and output
❑ Seizure precautions
❑ IV D5W/0.45% NS at 500 mL/8 hr
❑ Phenytoin (Dilantin) 2 mg/kg/min IV

❏ Diazapam (Valium) 0.3 mg/kg IV push given over 3 minutes every 15–30 min to a total dose of 10 mg, repeat every 2–4 hr for seizure activity following Dilantin administration

❏ Acetaminophen (Tylenol) 320 mg PO every 4 hours alternating with Ibuprofen 7.5 mg/kg PO every 6 hours

Identify the orders that require calculations.

Set up and solve each problem using dimensional analysis.

1. Calculate how many mL/hr to set the IV pump. Supply: D5W/0.45% NS 500 mL.

2. Calculate how many mL/hr to set the IV pump to administer Dilantin. Supply: dilantin 100 mg/50 mL to be administered over 15 minutes.

3. Calculate how many mL of diazepam will be given IV push over 3 minutes. Supply: diazepam 5 mg/mL.

4. Calculate how many mL of acetaminophen will be given every 4 hours PO. Supply: acetaminophen 100 mg/mL.

5. Calculate how many mL of ibuprofen will be given PO every 6 hours. Supply: ibuprofen 100 mg/5 mL.

■ CASE STUDY 28   *Fever of Unknown Origin*

A 10-year old child is admitted to the pediatric hospital with fever of unknown origin. The child's weight is 80 lb. The orders from the physician include:

❏ Admit to the Pediatric Unit
❏ Complete blood count with differential, chest x-ray, urinalysis, chemistry panel, and sputum culture
❏ Vitals every 4 hours
❏ Monitor intake and output
❏ Acetaminophen (Tylenol) 400 mg PO every 4 h alternating with ibuprofen 7.5 mg/kg PO every 6 h
❏ IV D5W/0.45% NS at 500 mL/4 hr
❏ Unasyn 1500 mg IV every 6 h

Identify the orders that require calculations.

Set up and solve each problem using dimensional analysis.

1. Calculate how many mL of acetaminophen will be given every 4 hours PO. Supply: acetaminophen 500 mg/15 mL.

2. Calculate how many mL of ibuprofen will be given every 6 h PO. Supply: ibuprofen 100 mg/5 mL.

3. Calculate how many mL/hr to set the IV pump. Supply: D5W/0.45% NS 500 mL.

4. Calculate the gtt/min using a microtubing (60 gtt/mL).

5. Calculate how many mL/hr to set the IV pump to administer Unasyn. Supply: Unasyn 1.5 g/50 mL over 30 minutes.

■ CASE STUDY 29   TURP with CBI

A 58-year-old male is admitted to the medical/surgical unit following surgery for transurethral resection of prostate. The physician's post-operative orders include:

❏ Admit to the medical/surgical unit
❏ Monitor intake and output
❏ Monitor urinary output hourly
❏ Vitals every 2 hr
❏ Monitor for symptoms of TURP Syndrome
❏ Adjust rate of continuous bladder irrigation 3 Liter bags of sterile normal saline to maintain a patent catheter, adjust rate to maintain pink to clear urine, and maintain urinary catheter traction
❏ IV D5W/0.45% normal saline 1000 mL/8 hr
❏ Ciprofloxacin (Cipro) 400 mg IV every 12 hr
❏ Docusate sodium (Colace) 100 mg PO bid
❏ Dimenhydrinate 25 mg IV every 4 hr prn
❏ Acetaminophen (Tylenol) 300 mg with 30 mg of codeine PO 1 to 2 tablets every 4 to 6 hr prn
❏ Discontinue IV when drinking well
❏ Complete blood count, electrolytes, creatinine in am

Identify the orders that require calculations.

Set up and solve each problem using dimensional analysis.

1. Calculate how many mL/hr to set the IV pump. Supply: D5W/0.45% NS 1000 mL bag.

2. Calculate how many gtt/min using 20 gtt/mL IV tubing.

3. Calculate how many mL/hr to set the IV pump to deliver the Cipro. Supply: Ciprofloxasin 400 mg/200 mL D5W to infuse over 60 minutes.

4. Calculate how many capsules to give of Colace. Supply: docusate sodium 100 mg/capsule.

5. Calculate how many mL will be given of dimenhydrinate.

■ CASE STUDY 30   **Hypercholesterolemia**

A 40-year-old male returns to his nurse practitioner's office after 3 months for a cholesterol level of 240 mg/dl. The nurse practitioner's orders include:

❏ Continue low-fat, high fiber diet
❏ Continue to briskly walk 3 to 4 times weekly for 30 minutes
❏ Stop smoking and begin Chantix 0.5 mg PO once daily for days 1–3 then 0.5 mg PO bid for Day 4–7, then 1 mg PO for day 8
❏ Atorvastatin (Lipitor) 20 mg PO daily
❏ Cholestyramine resin 4 g/dose PO bid to be taken 1 hr before Lipitor
❏ Niacin 1.5 g/day PO
❏ Return appointment in 4 weeks for lipid levels.

Identify the orders that require calculations.

Set up and solve each problem using dimensional analysis.

1. Calculate how many tablets of Chantix the patient will be taking on days 1–3. Supply: Chantix 0.5 mg tablets.

2. Calculate how many tablets of Chantix the patient will be taking on day 8. Supply: Chantix 0.5 mg tablets.

3. Calculate how many tablets of Lipitor the patient will be taking. Supply: Lipitor 10 mg tablets.

4. Calculate how many g/day of cholestyramine resin the patient will be taking. Supply: Cholestyramine resin 4 g/dose powder to be mixed with 4 to 6 oz of fluid.

5. Calculate how many tablets/day of niacin the patient is taking. Supply: Niacin 500 mg tablets.

■ CASE STUDY 31   **Hypertension**

A 60-year-old male returns to his nurse practitioner's office after 3 months for elevated blood pressure. Patient's weight: 90 kg. The nurse practitioner's orders include:

❏ Continue on low-sodium diet
❏ Continue to briskly walk 3 to 4 times weekly for 30 minutes
❏ Maintain a fluid intake of 2 L/day
❏ Nifedipine (Procardia XL) 60 mg PO once daily for 14 days then return to the office for re-evaluation
❏ Docusate sodium (Colace) 100 mg PO bid
❏ Hydrochlorothiazide (HydroDIURIL) 25 mg daily PO in am with a glass of orange juice
❏ Report any weight gain of greater than 2 lb/day
❏ Return appointment in 14 days for re-evaluation of blood pressure

Identify the orders that require calculations.

Set up and solve each problem using dimensional analysis.

1. Calculate how many mL/meal the patient will need to consume.

2. Calculate how many tablets of nifedipine the patient is taking. Supply: Procardia XL 30 mg/tablets.

3. Calculate how many capsules of docusate sodium the patient is taking. Supply: Colace 100 mg/capsule.

4. Calculate how many tablets of hydrochlorothiazide the patient is taking. Supply: HydroDIURIL 50 mg/tablets.

5. Calculate the weight gain from 90 kg to 95 kg that will be reported to the nurse practitioner in lb.

■ CASE STUDY 32   **Diabetic Ketoacidosis**

A 16-year-old is admitted to the medical intensive care unit with diabetic ketoacidosis secondary to fever. The patient weighs 125 lbs. The orders from the physician include:

- ❑ Admit to the medical intensive care unit
- ❑ Complete blood count, electrolytes, blood sugar, ABGs, and ECG
- ❑ Blood, urine, and sputum cultures
- ❑ Electrolytes and blood sugars hourly until stable
- ❑ Strict intake and output
- ❑ Daily weight
- ❑ Vitals hourly × 4 then every 2 hours × 4 then every 4 hr
- ❑ IV 0.9% NS 1000 mL/8 hr
- ❑ Regular insulin 0.15 units/kg IV bolus followed by the continuous intravenous infusion of regular insulin 0.1 unit/kg/hr in 0.9% NS
- ❑ Change IV fluids to D5W/0.45% NS when plasma glucose falls to under 250 mg/dL at 10 mL/kg/hr
- ❑ Ampicillin sodium 500 mg every 6 hr IVPB for 3 days

Identify the orders that require calculations.

Set up and solve each problem using dimensional analysis.

1. Calculate the mL/hr to set the IV pump to 1000 mL/8 hr. Supply: 0.9% NS 1000 mL.

2. Calculate the mL for the IV bolus to infuse regular insulin at 0.15 units/kg. Supply: 250 mL 0.9% NS with 250 units regular insulin.

3. Calculate the mL/hr to set the IV pump for the continuous infusion of regular insulin at 0.1 unit/kg/hr in 0.9% NS. Supply: 250 mL 0.9% NS with 250 units regular insulin.

4. Calculate the mL/hr to set the IV pump after the plasma glucose falls to under 250 mg/dL. Supply: D5W/0.45% NS 1000 mL

5. Calculate the mL/hr to set the IV pump to infuse ampicillin sodium. Supply: ampicillin sodium 1 g/100 mL over 30 min.

■ CASE STUDY 33   End-Stage Renal Failure

A 60-year-old patient is seen at the dialysis center for weekly dialysis treatment. The patient weighs 140 lbs after dialysis. The orders from the physician include:

❏ Obtain weight three times weekly prior to and after dialysis treatment
❏ Furosemide 120 mg PO bid
❏ Metolazone (Zaroxolyn) 10 mg PO daily
❏ Enalapril maleate (Vasotec) 2.5 mg PO bid
❏ Epogen 100 units/kg IV three times weekly in venous line following dialysis
❏ Calcium Carbonate 10 g/day in divided doses with meals

Identify the orders that require calculations.

Set up and solve each problem using dimensional analysis.

1. Calculate how many tablets of Furosemide the patient is taking. Supply: Furosemide 80 mg/tablets.

2. Calculate how many tablets of Zaroxolyn the patient is taking. Supply: Metolazone 5 mg/tablet.

3. Calculate how many tablets of Vasotec the patient is taking. Supply: Enalapril maleate 2.5 mg/tablets.

4. Calculate how many mL of Epogen the patient should receive three times weekly. Supply: Epogen 4,000 units/mL.

5. Calculate how many tablets/meal of calcium carbonate the patient will receive. Supply: calcium carbonate 1500 mg/tablets.

■ CASE STUDY 34   Fluid Volume Deficit

A five-year old child is admitted to the pediatric unit for fluid volume deficit secondary to gastroenteritis. The child's weight is 35 lb. The orders from the physician include:

❏ Admit to pediatric unit for 24-hour observation
❏ Monitor intake and output
❏ IV 50 mL/kg 0.9% NS/2.5% dextrose over 4 hr
❏ Discontinue IV when taking PO fluids without emesis
❏ Acetaminophen (Tylenol) 400 mg/dose PO every 4 hours alternating with ibuprofen 7.5 mg/kg PO every 6 hours

❏ Encourage sips of fluids every 10 minutes if not vomiting, repeated every 15 minutes until able to consume 30 mL then fluids as tolerated at 1.5 oz/lb/24 hr
❏ Pedialyte 53 oz/24 hr when tolerating fluids

Identify the orders that require calculations.

Set up and solve each problem using dimensional analysis.

1. Calculate the mL/hr to set the IV pump to infuse 50 mL/kg/4 hr. Supply: 1000 mL 0.9% NS/2.5% dextrose.

2. Calculate how many mL of acetaminophen will be given PO. Supply: acetaminophen 100 mg/mL solution.

3. Calculate how many mL of ibuprofen per dose will be given PO. Supply: ibuprofen 100 mg/5 mL solution.

4. Calculate how many mL/hr of fluids the child will receive.

5. Calculate how many mL/hr of pedialyte the child will receive.

■ CASE STUDY 35   **Increased Intracranial Pressure**

A 35-year-old male is admitted to the hospital with signs and symptoms of increased intracranial pressure secondary to brain metastasis. The patient weighs 75 kg. The orders from the physician include:

❏ Admit to oncology unit
❏ IV 0.9% NS 1000 mL/10 hr
❏ Loading dose of phenytoin (Dilantin) 10 mg/kg IV push (50 mg/min) then Dilantin 100 mg IV every 8 hr
❏ Mannitol 0.5 g/kg/10 min IV initial dose followed by Mannitol 0.25 g/kg IV every 4 hr
❏ Dexamethasone 10 mg IV
❏ Furosemide 0.5 mg/kg IV push
❏ Elevate HOB 25–30 degrees to promote intracranial drainage
❏ Bedrest in a quiet, darkened environment

Identify the orders that require calculations.

Set up and solve each problem using dimensional analysis.

1. Calculate the mL/hr to set the IV pump to infuse 0.9% NS. Supply: 1000 mL 0.9% NS.

2. Calculate how many mL of Dilantin the patient will receive as a loading dose. Supply: Dilantin 1000 mg/20 mL 0.9% NS.

3. Calculate the mL/hr to set the IV pump to infuse the Mannitol ordered every 4 h. Supply: Mannitol 100 g/500 mL D5W.

4. Calculate how many mL of dexamethasone will be given IV push. Supply: Decadron 120 mg/5 mL.

5. Calculate how many mL of furosemide will be given IV push. Supply: furosemide 10 mg/mL.

References

WebMD.com http://www.webmd.com/
Merck Manual online http://www.merck.com/mmpe/index.html
GlobalRPh.com http://www.globalrph.com/
PDR for Nurse's Drug Handbook (2007 edition).

ANSWER KEY FOR SECTION 3: CASE STUDIES

Case Study 1: Congestive Heart Failure

Orders requiring calculations: IV of D5W/$\frac{1}{2}$ NS at 50 mL/hr; weight gain; furosemide 40 mg IV every d; digoxin 0.125 mg PO qd; KCl 20 mEq PO tid

1. $\dfrac{50\ \text{mL}}{\text{hr}} \left| \dfrac{60\ \text{gtt}}{\text{mL}} \right| \dfrac{1\ \text{hr}}{60\ \text{min}} = \dfrac{50 \times 1}{60} = \dfrac{50\ \text{gtt}}{\text{min}}$

2. $\dfrac{10\ \text{lb}}{} \left| \dfrac{1\ \text{kg}}{2.2\ \text{lb}} \right| \dfrac{10 \times 1}{2.2} = \dfrac{10}{2.2} = 4.5\ \text{kg}$

3. $\dfrac{40\ \text{mg}}{} \left| \dfrac{\text{mL}}{10\ \text{mg}} \right| \dfrac{4}{1} = 4\ \text{mL}$

4. $\dfrac{0.125\ \text{mg}}{} \left| \dfrac{\text{tablet}}{0.25\ \text{mg}} \right| \dfrac{0.125}{0.25} = 0.5\ \text{tablet}$

5. $\dfrac{20\ \text{mEq}}{} \left| \dfrac{\text{tablet}}{10\ \text{mEq}} \right| \dfrac{2}{1} = 2\ \text{tablets}$

Case Study 2: COPD/Emphysema

Orders requiring calculations: IV of D5W/$\frac{1}{2}$ NS 1000 mL/8 hr; aminophylline IV loading dose of 5.6 mg/kg over 30 min followed by 0.5 mg/kg/hr continuous IV; erythromycin 800 mg IV every 6h; accurate intake/output.

1. $\dfrac{1000\ \text{mL}}{8\ \text{hr}} \left| \dfrac{1000}{8} = \dfrac{125\ \text{mL}}{\text{hr}} \right.$

2. $\dfrac{5.6\ \text{mg}}{\text{kg/30 min}} \left| \dfrac{100\ \text{mL}}{100\ \text{mg}} \right| \dfrac{1\ \text{kg}}{2.2\ \text{lb}} \left| 140\ \text{lb} \right| \dfrac{60\ \text{min}}{1\ \text{hr}} \ \dfrac{5.6 \times 14 \times 6}{3 \times 2.2}$

$\dfrac{470.4}{6.6} = \dfrac{71.3\ \text{mL}}{\text{hr}}\ \text{or}\ \dfrac{71\ \text{mL}}{\text{hr}}$

3. $\dfrac{0.5\ \text{mg}}{\text{kg/hr}} \left| \dfrac{250\ \text{mL}}{1\ \text{g}} \right| \dfrac{1\ \text{g}}{1000\ \text{mg}} \left| \dfrac{1\ \text{kg}}{2.2\ \text{lb}} \right| 140\ \text{lb} \left| \dfrac{0.5 \times 25 \times 1 \times 14}{10 \times 2.2} \right.$

$\dfrac{175}{22} = \dfrac{7.9\ \text{mL}}{\text{hr}}\ \text{or}\ \dfrac{8\ \text{mL}}{\text{hr}}$

4. $\dfrac{800\ \text{mg}}{} \left| \dfrac{20\ \text{mL}}{1\ \text{g}} \right| \dfrac{1\ \text{g}}{1000\ \text{mg}} \left| \dfrac{8 \times 2}{1} \right. = 16\ \text{mL}$

$\dfrac{266\ \text{mL}}{1\ \text{hr}} = \dfrac{266\ \text{mL}}{\text{hr}}$

5. $\dfrac{3\ \text{L}}{\text{day}} \left| \dfrac{\text{day}}{3\ \text{shifts}} \right| \dfrac{1000\ \text{mL}}{1\ \text{L}} \left| \dfrac{1000}{1} \right. = \dfrac{1000\ \text{mL}}{\text{shift}}$

Case Study 3: Small Cell Lung Cancer

Orders requiring calculations: IV D5W/$\frac{1}{2}$ NS 1000 mL with 10 mEq KCl at 125 mL/hr; Neupogen 5 mcg/kg SQ daily; gentamicin 80 mg IV every 8h; Decadron 8 mg IV daily; Fortaz 1 g IV every 8h

1. $\dfrac{125\ \text{mL}}{\text{hr}} \left| \dfrac{20\ \text{gtt}}{\text{mL}} \right| \dfrac{1\ \text{hr}}{60\ \text{min}} \left| \dfrac{125 \times 2 \times 1}{6} \right| \dfrac{250}{6} = \dfrac{41.6\ \text{or}\ 42\ \text{gtt}}{\text{min}}$

2. $\dfrac{5\ \text{mcg}}{\text{kg}} \left| \dfrac{1\ \text{kg}}{2.2\ \text{lb}} \right| 160\ \text{lb} \left| \dfrac{5 \times 1 \times 160}{2.2} \right| \dfrac{800}{2.2} = 363.6\ \text{mcg or}\ 364\ \text{mcg}$

3. $\dfrac{80\ \text{mg}}{} \left| \dfrac{\text{mL}}{40\ \text{mg}} \right| \dfrac{8}{4} = 2\ \text{mL}$

$\dfrac{102\ \text{mL}}{1\ \text{hr}} = \dfrac{102\ \text{mL}}{\text{hr}}$

4. $\dfrac{8\ \text{mg}}{} \left| \dfrac{\text{mL}}{4\ \text{mg}} \right| \dfrac{8}{4} = 2\ \text{mL}$

5. $\dfrac{50\ \text{mL}}{30\ \text{min}} \left| \dfrac{60\ \text{min}}{1\ \text{hr}} \right| \dfrac{50 \times 6}{3 \times 1} \left| \dfrac{300}{3} \right. = \dfrac{100\ \text{mL}}{\text{hr}}$

Case Study 4: Acquired Immunodeficiency Syndrome (AIDS)

Orders requiring calculations: IV D5W/$\frac{1}{2}$ NS at 150 mL/hr; acyclovir 350 mg IV every 8h; Neupogen 300 mcg SQ daily; Epogen 100 units/kg SQ three times a week; vancomycin 800 mg IV every 6h

1.
$$\frac{150 \text{ mL}}{\text{hr}} \left| \frac{20 \text{ gtt}}{\text{mL}} \right| \frac{1 \text{ hr}}{60 \text{ min}} \left| \frac{150 \times 2 \times 1}{6} \right| \frac{300}{6} = \frac{50 \text{ gtt}}{\text{min}}$$

2.
$$\frac{350 \text{ mg}}{} \left| \frac{10 \text{ mL}}{500 \text{ mg}} \right| \frac{35 \times 1}{5} \left| \frac{35}{5} \right. = 7 \text{ mL}$$

$$\frac{107 \text{ mL}}{1 \text{ hr}} \left| \frac{107}{1} \right. = \frac{107 \text{ mL}}{\text{hr}}$$

3.
$$\frac{300 \text{ mcg}}{} \left| \frac{1 \text{ mL}}{300 \text{ mcg}} \right. = 1 \text{ mL}$$

4.
$$\frac{100 \text{ units}}{\text{kg}} \left| \frac{\text{mL}}{4000 \text{ units}} \right| \frac{1 \text{ kg}}{2.2 \text{ lb}} \left| \frac{100 \text{ lb}}{} \right| \frac{10 \times 1 \times 1}{4 \times 2.2} \left| \frac{10}{8.8} \right. = 1.1 \text{ mL or 1 mL}$$

5.
$$\frac{800 \text{ mg}}{} \left| \frac{10 \text{ mL}}{1 \text{ g}} \right| \frac{1 \text{ g}}{1000 \text{ mg}} \left| \frac{80 \times 1}{10} \right| \frac{80}{10} = 8 \text{ mL}$$

$$\frac{108 \text{ mL}}{60 \text{ min}} \left| \frac{60 \text{ min}}{1 \text{ hr}} \right| \frac{108}{1} = \frac{108 \text{ mL}}{\text{hr}}$$

Case Study 5: Sickle Cell Anemia

Orders requiring calculations: IV D5W/$\frac{1}{2}$ NS at 150 mL/hr; Zofran 8 mg IV every 8h; morphine sulfate 5 mg IV prn; Hydrea 10 mg/kg/day PO; folic acid 0.5 mg daily PO

1.
$$\frac{150 \text{ mL}}{\text{hr}} \left| \frac{10 \text{ gtt}}{\text{mL}} \right| \frac{1 \text{ hr}}{60 \text{ min}} \left| \frac{150 \times 1 \times 1}{6} \right| \frac{150}{6} = \frac{25 \text{ gtt}}{\text{min}}$$

2.
$$\frac{50 \text{ mL}}{15 \text{ min}} \left| \frac{60 \text{ min}}{1 \text{ hr}} \right| \frac{50 \times 60}{15 \times 1} \left| \frac{3000}{15} \right. = \frac{200 \text{ mL}}{\text{hr}}$$

3.
$$\frac{5 \text{ mg}}{} \left| \frac{\text{mL}}{10 \text{ mg}} \right| \frac{5}{10} = 0.5 \text{ mL}$$

4.
$$\frac{10 \text{ mg}}{\text{kg day}} \left| \frac{1 \text{ kg}}{2.2 \text{ lb}} \right| \frac{125 \text{ lb}}{} \left| \frac{10 \times 1 \times 125}{2.2} \right| \frac{1250}{2.2} = \frac{568 \text{ mg}}{\text{day}}$$

5.
$$\frac{0.5 \text{ mg}}{} \left| \frac{\text{tablet}}{1 \text{ mg}} \right| \frac{0.5}{1} = 0.5 \text{ tablet}$$

Case Study 6: Deep Vein Thrombosis

Orders requiring calculations: IV D5W/$\frac{1}{2}$ NS with 20 mEq KCl at 50 mL/hr; heparin 5000 units IV push followed by continuous IV infusion of 1000 units/hr; Lasix 20 mg IV bid; morphine 5 mg IV every 4h

1.
$$\frac{50 \text{ mL}}{\text{hr}} \left| \frac{60 \text{ gtt}}{\text{mL}} \right| \frac{1 \text{ hr}}{60 \text{ min}} \left| \frac{50 \times 1}{60} \right| \frac{50}{} = \frac{50 \text{ gtt}}{\text{min}}$$

2.
$$\frac{5000 \text{ units}}{} \left| \frac{\text{mL}}{10,000 \text{ units}} \right| \frac{5}{10} = 0.5 \text{ mL}$$

3.
$$\frac{1000 \text{ units}}{\text{hr}} \left| \frac{250 \text{ mL}}{25,000 \text{ units}} \right| \frac{10}{} = \frac{10 \text{ mL}}{\text{hr}}$$

4.
$$\frac{20 \text{ mg}}{} \left| \frac{\text{mL}}{10 \text{ mg}} \right| \frac{2}{1} = 2 \text{ mL}$$

5.
$$\frac{5 \text{ mg}}{} \left| \frac{\text{mL}}{10 \text{ mg}} \right| \frac{5}{10} = 0.5 \text{ mL}$$

Case Study 7: Bone Marrow Transplant

Orders requiring calculations: IV D5W/$\frac{1}{2}$ NS with 20 mEq KCl/L at 80 mL/hr; Fortaz 2 g IV every 8h; vancomycin 1 g IV every 6h; Claforan 1 g IV every 12h; erythromycin 800 mg IV every 6h

1.
$$\frac{80 \text{ mL}}{\text{hr}} \left| \frac{20 \text{ mEq}}{1 \text{ L}} \right| \frac{1 \text{ L}}{1000 \text{ mL}} \left| \frac{8 \times 2}{10} \right| \frac{16}{10} = \frac{1.6 \text{ mEq}}{\text{hr}}$$

2. $\dfrac{\cancel{2}\text{ g} \mid 10\,\text{(mL)} \mid 10}{\cancel{2}\text{ g}} = 10\text{ mL}$

$\dfrac{60\,\text{(mL)} \mid 60\,\cancel{\text{min}} \mid 60 \times 6 \mid 360}{30\,\cancel{\text{min}} \mid 1\,\text{(hr)} \mid 3 \times 1 \mid 3} = 120\,\dfrac{\text{mL}}{\text{hr}}$

3. $\dfrac{\cancel{1}\text{ g} \mid 10\,\text{(mL)} \mid 1000\,\cancel{\text{mg}} \mid 10 \times 10 \mid 100}{500\,\cancel{\text{mg}} \mid \cancel{1}\text{ g} \mid 5 \mid 5} = 20\text{ mL}$

$\dfrac{120\,\text{(mL)} \mid 60\,\cancel{\text{min}} \mid 120}{60\,\cancel{\text{min}} \mid 1\,\text{(hr)} \mid 1} = 120\,\dfrac{\text{mL}}{\text{hr}}$

4. $\dfrac{\cancel{1}\text{ g} \mid 4\,\text{(mL)} \mid 1000\,\cancel{\text{mg}} \mid 4 \times 10 \mid 40}{600\,\cancel{\text{mg}} \mid \cancel{1}\text{ g} \mid 6 \mid 6} = 6.7\text{ mL or }7\text{ mL}$

$\dfrac{107\,\text{(mL)} \mid 107}{1\,\text{(hr)} \mid 1} = 107\,\dfrac{\text{mL}}{\text{hr}}$

5. $\dfrac{800\,\cancel{\text{mg}} \mid 20\,\text{(mL)} \mid \cancel{1}\text{ g} \mid 8 \times 2 \mid 16}{\cancel{1}\text{ g} \mid 1000\,\cancel{\text{mg}} \mid 1 \mid 1} = 16\text{ mL}$

$\dfrac{266\,\text{(mL)} \mid 60\,\cancel{\text{min}} \mid 266}{60\,\cancel{\text{min}} \mid 1\,\text{(hr)} \mid 1} = 266\,\dfrac{\text{mL}}{\text{hr}}$

Case Study 8: Pneumonia

Orders requiring calculations: Clindamycin 400 mg IV every 6h; guaifenesin 200 mg PO every 4h; terbutaline 2.5 mg PO tid; MS Contin 30 mg PO every 4h prn

1. $\dfrac{400\,\cancel{\text{mg}} \mid 4\,\text{(mL)} \mid 4 \times 4 \mid 16}{600\,\cancel{\text{mg}} \mid 6 \mid 6} = 2.7\text{ mL or }3\text{ mL}$

$\dfrac{53\,\text{(mL)} \mid 53}{\text{(hr)}} = 53\,\dfrac{\text{mL}}{\text{hr}}$

2. $\dfrac{53\,\cancel{\text{mL}} \mid 20\,\text{(gtt)} \mid 1\,\cancel{\text{hr}} \mid 53 \times 2 \times 1 \mid 106}{\cancel{\text{hr}} \mid \cancel{\text{mL}} \mid 60\,\text{(min)} \mid 6 \mid 6} = 18\,\dfrac{\text{gtt}}{\text{min}}$

3. $\dfrac{200\,\cancel{\text{mg}} \mid \cancel{\text{tsp}} \mid 5\,\text{(mL)} \mid 20 \times 5 \mid 100}{30\,\cancel{\text{mg}} \mid 1\,\cancel{\text{tsp}} \mid 3 \times 1 \mid 3} = 33\text{ mL}$

4. $\dfrac{2.5\,\cancel{\text{mg}} \mid \text{(tablet)} \mid 2.5}{5\,\cancel{\text{mg}} \mid 5} = 0.5\text{ tablet}$

5. $\dfrac{30\,\cancel{\text{mg}} \mid \text{(tablet)} \mid 30}{30\,\cancel{\text{mg}} \mid 30} = 1\text{ tablet}$

Case Study 9: Pain

Orders requiring calculations: IV D5W/$\frac{1}{2}$ NS with 20 mEq KCl/L at 60 mL/hr; IV 500 mL NS with 25 mg dilaudid and 50 mg thorazine at 21 mL/hr; Bumex 2 mg IV every AM after albumin infusion

1. $\dfrac{60\,\cancel{\text{mL}} \mid 20\,\text{(mEq)} \mid \cancel{1}\text{ L} \mid 6 \times 2 \mid 12}{\text{(hr)} \mid \cancel{1}\text{ L} \mid 1000\,\cancel{\text{mL}} \mid 10 \mid 10} = 1.2\,\dfrac{\text{mEq}}{\text{hr}}$

2. $\dfrac{21\,\cancel{\text{mL}} \mid 25\,\text{(mg)} \mid 21 \times 25 \mid 525}{\text{(hr)} \mid 500\,\cancel{\text{mL}} \mid 500 \mid 500} = 1.05\,\dfrac{\text{mg}}{\text{hr}}$

3. $\dfrac{21\,\cancel{\text{mL}} \mid 50\,\text{(mg)} \mid 21 \times 5 \mid 105}{\text{(hr)} \mid 500\,\cancel{\text{mL}} \mid 50 \mid 50} = 2.1\,\dfrac{\text{mg}}{\text{hr}}$

4. $\dfrac{11\,\cancel{\text{mL}} \mid 25,000\,\text{(units)} \mid 11 \times 2500 \mid 27,500}{\text{(hr)} \mid 250\,\cancel{\text{mL}} \mid 25 \mid 25} = 1100\,\dfrac{\text{units}}{\text{hr}}$

5. $\dfrac{2\,\cancel{\text{mg}} \mid \text{(mL)} \mid 2}{0.25\,\cancel{\text{mg}} \mid 0.25} = 8\text{ mL}$

Case Study 10: Cirrhosis

Orders requiring calculations: IV D5W/$\frac{1}{2}$ NS with 20 mEq KCl at 125 mL/hr; IV Zantac 150 mg/250 mL NS at 11 mL/hr; vitamin K 10 mg SQ every AM; Spironolactone 50 mg PO bid; Lasix 80 mg IV every AM

1. $\dfrac{125\,\cancel{\text{mL}} \mid 20\,\text{(gtt)} \mid 1\,\cancel{\text{hr}} \mid 125 \times 2 \times 1 \mid 250}{\cancel{\text{hr}} \mid \cancel{\text{mL}} \mid 60\,\text{(min)} \mid 6 \mid 6} = 41.66\text{ or }42\,\dfrac{\text{gtt}}{\text{min}}$

2. $\dfrac{11\ \cancel{mL}}{\cancel{hr}} \Big| \dfrac{15\theta\ \cancel{mg}}{25\theta\ \cancel{mL}} \Big| \dfrac{11 \times 15}{25} \Big| \dfrac{165}{25} = 6.6\ \dfrac{mg}{hr}$

3. $\dfrac{10\ \cancel{mg}}{} \Big| \dfrac{\cancel{mL}}{10\ \cancel{mg}} \Big| \dfrac{10}{10} = 1\ mL$

4. $\dfrac{50\ \cancel{mg}}{} \Big| \dfrac{\text{tablet}}{25\ \cancel{mg}} \Big| \dfrac{50}{25} = 2\ tablets$

5. $\dfrac{8\theta\ \cancel{mg}}{} \Big| \dfrac{\cancel{mL}}{1\theta\ \cancel{mg}} \Big| \dfrac{8}{1} = 8\ mL$

Case Study 11: Hyperemesis Gravidarum

Orders requiring calculations: IV D5½ NS at 150 mL/hr and 100 mL/hr; droperidol (Inapsine) 1 mg IV; metoclopramide (Reglan) 20 mg IV in 50 mL of D5W to infuse over 15 min; diphenhydramine (Benadryl) 25 mg; dexamethasone (Decadron) 4 mg IV

1. $\dfrac{150\ \cancel{mL}}{\cancel{hr}} \Big| \dfrac{2\theta\ \text{gtt}}{\cancel{mL}} \Big| \dfrac{1\ \cancel{hr}}{6\theta\ \text{min}} \Big| \dfrac{150 \times 2 \times 1}{6} \Big| \dfrac{300}{6} = 50\ \dfrac{\text{gtt}}{\text{min}}$

$\dfrac{100\ \cancel{mL}}{\cancel{hr}} \Big| \dfrac{2\theta\ \text{gtt}}{\cancel{mL}} \Big| \dfrac{1\ \cancel{hr}}{6\theta\ \text{min}} \Big| \dfrac{100 \times 2 \times 1}{6} \Big| \dfrac{200}{6} = 33.3\ \text{or}\ 33\ \dfrac{\text{gtt}}{\text{min}}$

2. $\dfrac{1\ \cancel{mg}}{} \Big| \dfrac{\cancel{mL}}{2.5\ \cancel{mg}} \Big| \dfrac{1}{2.5} = 0.4\ mL$

3. $\dfrac{50\ \text{mL}}{15\ \cancel{min}} \Big| \dfrac{60\ \cancel{min}}{1\ \text{hr}} \Big| \dfrac{50 \times 60}{15 \times 1} \Big| \dfrac{3000}{15} = 200\ \dfrac{mL}{hr}$

4. $\dfrac{25\ \cancel{mg}}{} \Big| \dfrac{\cancel{mL}}{10\ \cancel{mg}} \Big| \dfrac{25}{10} = 2.5\ mL$

5. $\dfrac{4\ \cancel{mg}}{} \Big| \dfrac{\text{mL}}{4\ \cancel{mg}} \Big| \dfrac{4}{4} = 1\ mL$

Case Study 12: Preeclampsia

Orders requiring calculations: Methyldopa (Aldomet) 250 mg; Hydralazine (Apresoline) 5 mg IV; magnesium sulfate 4 g in 250 mL D5W loading dose to infuse over 30 min; magnesium sulfate 40 g in 1000 mL LR to infuse at 1 g/hr; nifedipine (Procardia) 10 mg sublingual

1. $\dfrac{25\theta\ \cancel{mg}}{} \Big| \dfrac{\text{tablet}}{50\theta\ \cancel{mg}} \Big| \dfrac{25}{50} = 0.5\ tablets$

2. $\dfrac{5\ \cancel{mg}}{} \Big| \dfrac{\text{mL}}{20\ \cancel{mg}} \Big| \dfrac{5}{20} = 0.25\ mL$

3. $\dfrac{250\ \text{mL}}{3\theta\ \cancel{min}} \Big| \dfrac{6\theta\ \cancel{min}}{1\ \text{hr}} \Big| \dfrac{250 \times 6}{3 \times 1} \Big| \dfrac{1500}{3} = 500\ \dfrac{mL}{hr}$

4. $\dfrac{1\ \cancel{g}}{\text{hr}} \Big| \dfrac{100\theta\ \text{mL}}{4\theta\ \cancel{g}} \Big| \dfrac{1 \times 100}{4} \Big| \dfrac{100}{4} = 25\ \dfrac{mL}{hr}$

5. $\dfrac{10\ \cancel{mg}}{} \Big| \dfrac{\text{capsule}}{10\ \cancel{mg}} \Big| \dfrac{10}{10} = 1\ capsule$

Case Study 13: Premature Labor

Orders requiring calculations: Magnesium sulfate at 2 g/hr; terbutaline (Brethine) 0.25 mg SQ; nifedipine (Procardia) 20 mg; betamethasone 12 mg IM; LR 1000 mL over 8 hr

1. $\dfrac{250\ \text{mL}}{2\theta\ \cancel{min}} \Big| \dfrac{6\theta\ \cancel{min}}{1\ \text{hr}} \Big| \dfrac{250 \times 6}{2 \times 1} \Big| \dfrac{1500}{2} = 750\ \dfrac{mL}{hr}$

$\dfrac{2\ \cancel{g}}{\text{hr}} \Big| \dfrac{250\ \text{mL}}{4\ \cancel{g}} \Big| \dfrac{2 \times 250}{4} \Big| \dfrac{500}{4} = 125\ \dfrac{mL}{hr}$

2. $\dfrac{0.25\ \cancel{mg}}{} \Big| \dfrac{\text{mL}}{1\ \cancel{mg}} \Big| \dfrac{0.25}{1} = 0.25\ mL$

3. $\dfrac{2\theta\ \cancel{mg}}{} \Big| \dfrac{\text{capsule}}{1\theta\ \cancel{mg}} \Big| \dfrac{2}{1} = 2\ capsules$

4. $\dfrac{12\ \text{mg}}{}\ \bigg|\ \dfrac{\text{mL}}{6\ \text{mg}}\ \bigg|\ \dfrac{12}{6} = 2\ \text{mL}$

5. $\dfrac{1000\ \text{mL}}{8\ \text{hr}}\ \bigg|\ \dfrac{1000}{8} = 125\ \dfrac{\text{mL}}{\text{hr}}$

Case Study 14: Cystic Fibrosis

Orders requiring calculations: IV 0.9% normal saline at 75 mL/hr; Tagamet 30 mg PO; clindamycin 10 mg/kg IV; terbutaline 2.5 mg PO; tobramycin 1.5 mg/kg IV

1. $\dfrac{75\ \text{mL}}{\text{hr}}\ \bigg|\ \dfrac{15\ \text{gtt}}{\text{mL}}\ \bigg|\ \dfrac{1\ \text{hr}}{60\ \text{min}}\ \bigg|\ \dfrac{75\times15\times1}{60}\ \bigg|\ \dfrac{1125}{60} = 18.75\ \text{or}\ 19\ \dfrac{\text{gtt}}{\text{min}}$

2. $\dfrac{30\ \text{mg}}{\text{kg/day}}\ \bigg|\ \dfrac{\text{tablet}}{200\ \text{mg}}\ \bigg|\ \dfrac{1\ \text{kg}}{2.2\ \text{lb}}\ \bigg|\ \dfrac{65\ \text{lb}}{4\ \text{doses}}\ \bigg|\ \dfrac{\text{day}}{}\ \bigg|\ \dfrac{3\times1\times65}{20\times2.2\times4}\ \bigg|\ \dfrac{195}{176} = 1.1\ \text{or}\ 1\ \dfrac{\text{tablet}}{\text{dose}}$

3. $\dfrac{10\ \text{mg}}{\text{kg}}\ \bigg|\ \dfrac{1\ \text{kg}}{2.2\ \text{lb}}\ \bigg|\ \dfrac{65\ \text{lb}}{}\ \bigg|\ \dfrac{10\times1\times65}{2.2}\ \bigg|\ \dfrac{650}{2.2} = 295.45\ \text{or}\ 295\ \text{mg}$

$\dfrac{295\ \text{mg}}{}\ \bigg|\ \dfrac{\text{mL}}{150\ \text{mg}}\ \bigg|\ \dfrac{295}{150} = 1.96\ \text{or}\ 2\ \text{mL}$

$\dfrac{52\ \text{mL}}{20\ \text{min}}\ \bigg|\ \dfrac{60\ \text{min}}{1\ \text{hr}}\ \bigg|\ \dfrac{52\times6}{2\times1}\ \bigg|\ \dfrac{312}{2} = 156\ \dfrac{\text{mL}}{\text{hr}}$

4. $\dfrac{2.5\ \text{mg}}{}\ \bigg|\ \dfrac{\text{tablet}}{2.5\ \text{mg}}\ \bigg|\ \dfrac{2.5}{2.5} = 1\ \text{tablet}$

5. $\dfrac{1.5\ \text{mg}}{\text{kg}}\ \bigg|\ \dfrac{1\ \text{kg}}{2.2\ \text{lb}}\ \bigg|\ \dfrac{65\ \text{lb}}{}\ \bigg|\ \dfrac{1.5\times1\times65}{2.2}\ \bigg|\ \dfrac{97.5}{2.2} = 44.31\ \text{or}\ 44\ \text{mg}$

$\dfrac{44\ \text{mg}}{}\ \bigg|\ \dfrac{\text{mL}}{40\ \text{mg}}\ \bigg|\ \dfrac{44}{40} = 1.1\ \text{or}\ 1\ \text{mL}$

$\dfrac{51\ \text{mL}}{30\ \text{min}}\ \bigg|\ \dfrac{60\ \text{min}}{1\ \text{hr}}\ \bigg|\ \dfrac{51\times6}{3\times1}\ \bigg|\ \dfrac{306}{3} = 102\ \dfrac{\text{mL}}{\text{hr}}$

Case Study 15: Respiratory Syncytial Virus (RSV)

Orders requiring calculations: Acetaminophen elixir 120 mg PO; aminophylline 5 mg/kg to infuse over 30 min and 0.8 mg/kg/hr IV; RespiGam 750 mg/kg IV; Pediapred 1.5 mg/kg/day in three divided doses PO; ampicillin 100 mg/kg/day in divided doses every 6h IV

1. $\dfrac{120\ \text{mg}}{}\ \bigg|\ \dfrac{5\ \text{mL}}{120\ \text{mg}}\ \bigg|\ \dfrac{5}{} = 5\ \text{mL}$

2. $\dfrac{5\ \text{mg}}{\text{kg}}\ \bigg|\ \dfrac{1\ \text{kg}}{2.2\ \text{lb}}\ \bigg|\ \dfrac{30\ \text{lb}}{}\ \bigg|\ \dfrac{5\times1\times30}{2.2}\ \bigg|\ \dfrac{150}{2.2} = 68.18\ \text{or}\ 68.2\ \text{mg}$

$\dfrac{68.2\ \text{mg}}{30\ \text{min}}\ \bigg|\ \dfrac{100\ \text{mL}}{250\ \text{mg}}\ \bigg|\ \dfrac{60\ \text{min}}{1\ \text{hr}}\ \bigg|\ \dfrac{68.2\times10\times6}{3\times25\times1}\ \bigg|\ \dfrac{4092}{75} = 54.56\ \text{or}\ 54.6\ \dfrac{\text{mL}}{\text{hr}}$

$\dfrac{0.8\ \text{mg}}{\text{kg/hr}}\ \bigg|\ \dfrac{100\ \text{mL}}{250\ \text{mg}}\ \bigg|\ \dfrac{1\ \text{kg}}{2.2\ \text{lb}}\ \bigg|\ \dfrac{30\ \text{lb}}{}\ \bigg|\ \dfrac{0.8\times100\times1\times3}{25\times2.2}\ \bigg|\ \dfrac{240}{55} = 4.36\ \text{or}\ 4.4\ \dfrac{\text{mL}}{\text{hr}}$

3. $\dfrac{750\ \text{mg}}{\text{kg}}\ \bigg|\ \dfrac{1\ \text{kg}}{2.2\ \text{lb}}\ \bigg|\ \dfrac{30\ \text{lb}}{}\ \bigg|\ \dfrac{750\times1\times30}{2.2}\ \bigg|\ \dfrac{22{,}500}{2.2} = 10{,}227.27\ \text{or}\ 10{,}227.3\ \text{mg}$

4. $\dfrac{1.5\ \text{mg}}{\text{kg/day}}\ \bigg|\ \dfrac{5\ \text{mL}}{15\ \text{mg}}\ \bigg|\ \dfrac{1\ \text{kg}}{2.2\ \text{lb}}\ \bigg|\ \dfrac{30\ \text{lb}}{3\ \text{doses}}\ \bigg|\ \dfrac{\text{day}}{}\ \bigg|\ \dfrac{1.5\times5\times1\times30}{15\times2.2\times3}\ \bigg|\ \dfrac{225}{99} = 2.27\ \text{or}\ 2.3\ \dfrac{\text{mL}}{\text{dose}}$

5. $\dfrac{100\ \text{mg}}{\text{kg/day}}\ \bigg|\ \dfrac{1\ \text{kg}}{2.2\ \text{lb}}\ \bigg|\ \dfrac{30\ \text{lb}}{4\ \text{doses}}\ \bigg|\ \dfrac{\text{day}}{}\ \bigg|\ \dfrac{100\times1\times30}{2.2\times4}\ \bigg|\ \dfrac{3000}{8.8} = 340.9\ \text{or}\ 341\ \dfrac{\text{mg}}{\text{dose}}$

$\dfrac{341\ \text{mg}}{1\ \text{g}}\ \bigg|\ \dfrac{10\ \text{mL}}{1000\ \text{mg}}\ \bigg|\ \dfrac{1\ \text{g}}{1\times100}\ \bigg|\ \dfrac{341\times1\times1}{100}\ \bigg|\ \dfrac{341}{100} = 3.41\ \text{or}\ 3.4\ \text{mL}$

$\dfrac{53\ \text{mL}}{30\ \text{min}}\ \bigg|\ \dfrac{60\ \text{min}}{1\ \text{hr}}\ \bigg|\ \dfrac{53\times6}{3\times1}\ \bigg|\ \dfrac{318}{3} = 106\ \dfrac{\text{mL}}{\text{hr}}$

Case Study 16: Leukemia

Orders requiring calculations: IV D5W/NS with 20 mEq KCl 1000 mL over 8 h; allopurinol 200 mg PO; Fortaz 1 g IV; aztreonam 2 g IV; Flagyl 500 mg IV

1. $\dfrac{1000 \text{ mL}}{8 \text{ hr}} \bigg| \dfrac{1000}{8} = \dfrac{125 \text{ mL}}{\text{hr}}$

2. $\dfrac{200 \text{ mg}}{} \bigg| \dfrac{\text{tablet}}{100 \text{ mg}} \bigg| \dfrac{2}{1} = 2 \text{ tablets}$

3. $\dfrac{1 \text{ g}}{} \bigg| \dfrac{10 \text{ mL}}{1 \text{ g}} = 10 \text{ mL}$

$\dfrac{60 \text{ mL}}{30 \text{ min}} \bigg| \dfrac{60 \text{ min}}{1 \text{ hr}} \bigg| \dfrac{60 \times 6}{3 \times 1} \bigg| \dfrac{360}{3} = \dfrac{120 \text{ mL}}{\text{hr}}$

4. $\dfrac{2 \text{ g}}{} \bigg| \dfrac{10 \text{ mL}}{2 \text{ g}} = 10 \text{ mL}$

$\dfrac{110 \text{ mL}}{60 \text{ min}} \bigg| \dfrac{60 \text{ min}}{1 \text{ hr}} \bigg| \dfrac{110}{1} = \dfrac{110 \text{ mL}}{\text{hr}}$

5. $\dfrac{500 \text{ mg}}{1 \text{ hr}} \bigg| \dfrac{100 \text{ mL}}{500 \text{ mg}} \bigg| \dfrac{100}{1} = \dfrac{100 \text{ mL}}{\text{hr}}$

Case Study 17: Sepsis

Orders requiring calculations: NG breast milk with sterile water 120 mL per feeding; IV D10 and 20% lipids 120 mL/kg/day; aminophylline 5 mg/kg IV every 6h; cefotaxime 50 mg/kg every 12h; vancomycin 10 mg/kg/dose every 12h

1. $\dfrac{120 \text{ mL}}{\text{day}} \bigg| \dfrac{\text{day}}{24 \text{ hr}} \bigg| \dfrac{3 \text{ hr}}{\text{feeding}} \bigg| \dfrac{120 \times 3}{24} \bigg| \dfrac{360}{24} = \dfrac{15 \text{ mL}}{\text{feeding}}$

2. $\dfrac{120 \text{ mL}}{\text{kg/day}} \bigg| \dfrac{\text{day}}{24 \text{ hr}} \bigg| \dfrac{1 \text{ kg}}{1000 \text{ g}} \bigg| \dfrac{2005 \text{ g}}{} \bigg| \dfrac{12 \times 1 \times 2005}{24 \times 100} \bigg| \dfrac{24,060}{2400} = 10.025 \text{ or } \dfrac{10 \text{ mL}}{\text{hr}}$

3. $\dfrac{5 \text{ mg}}{\text{kg}} \bigg| \dfrac{1 \text{ kg}}{1000 \text{ g}} \bigg| \dfrac{2005 \text{ g}}{} \bigg| \dfrac{5 \times 1 \times 2005}{1000} \bigg| \dfrac{10025}{1000} = 10.025 \text{ or } 10 \text{ mg}$

$\dfrac{10 \text{ mg}}{5 \text{ min}} \bigg| \dfrac{10 \text{ mL}}{50 \text{ mg}} \bigg| \dfrac{60 \text{ min}}{1 \text{ hr}} \bigg| \dfrac{10 \times 10 \times 6}{5 \times 5 \times 1} \bigg| \dfrac{600}{25} = \dfrac{24 \text{ mL}}{\text{hr}}$

4. $\dfrac{50 \text{ mg}}{\text{kg}} \bigg| \dfrac{1 \text{ kg}}{1000 \text{ g}} \bigg| \dfrac{2005 \text{ g}}{} \bigg| \dfrac{5 \times 1 \times 2005}{100} \bigg| \dfrac{10025}{100} = 100.25 \text{ or } 100 \text{ mg}$

$\dfrac{100 \text{ mg}}{30 \text{ min}} \bigg| \dfrac{\text{mL}}{40 \text{ mg}} \bigg| \dfrac{60 \text{ min}}{1 \text{ hr}} \bigg| \dfrac{10 \times 6}{3 \times 4 \times 1} \bigg| \dfrac{60}{12} = \dfrac{5 \text{ mL}}{\text{hr}}$

5. $\dfrac{10 \text{ mg}}{\text{kg/dose}} \bigg| \dfrac{1 \text{ kg}}{1000 \text{ g}} \bigg| \dfrac{2005 \text{ g}}{} \bigg| \dfrac{1 \times 1 \times 2005}{100} \bigg| \dfrac{2005}{100} = 20.05 \text{ or } \dfrac{20 \text{ mg}}{\text{dose}}$

$\dfrac{20 \text{ mg}}{1 \text{ hr}} \bigg| \dfrac{1 \text{ mL}}{5 \text{ mg}} \bigg| \dfrac{20 \times 1}{1 \times 5} \bigg| \dfrac{20}{5} = \dfrac{4 \text{ mL}}{\text{hr}}$

Case Study 18: Bronchopulmonary Dysplasia

Orders requiring calculations: NG feedings with Special Care with Iron 120 KCal/kg/day; chlorothiazide 10 mg/kg/day; Fer-In-Sol 2 mg/kg/day; vitamin E 25 units/kg/day in divided doses every 12h; caffeine citrate 5 mg/kg/dose daily

1. $\dfrac{120 \text{ kcal}}{\text{kg/day}} \bigg| \dfrac{1 \text{ kg}}{1000 \text{ g}} \bigg| \dfrac{996 \text{ g}}{} \bigg| \dfrac{12 \times 1 \times 996}{100} \bigg| \dfrac{11,952}{100} = 119.52 \text{ or } \dfrac{120 \text{ kcal}}{\text{day}}$

$\dfrac{120 \text{ kcal}}{\text{day}} \bigg| \dfrac{\text{oz}}{24 \text{ kcal}} \bigg| \dfrac{30 \text{ mL}}{1 \text{ oz}} \bigg| \dfrac{120 \times 30}{24 \times 1} \bigg| \dfrac{3600}{24} = \dfrac{150 \text{ mL}}{\text{day}}$

2. $\dfrac{10 \text{ mg}}{\text{kg/day}} \bigg| \dfrac{1 \text{ kg}}{1000 \text{ g}} \bigg| \dfrac{996 \text{ g}}{} \bigg| \dfrac{1 \times 1 \times 996}{100} \bigg| \dfrac{996}{100} = 9.96 \text{ or } \dfrac{10 \text{ mg}}{\text{day}}$

$\dfrac{10 \text{ mg}}{\text{day}} \bigg| \dfrac{5 \text{ mL}}{250 \text{ mg}} \bigg| \dfrac{1 \times 5}{25} \bigg| \dfrac{5}{25} = \dfrac{0.2 \text{ mL}}{\text{day}}$

3. $\dfrac{2 \text{ mg}}{\text{kg/day}} \bigg| \dfrac{1 \text{ kg}}{1000 \text{ g}} \bigg| \dfrac{996 \text{ g}}{} \bigg| \dfrac{2 \times 1 \times 996}{1000} \bigg| \dfrac{1992}{1000} = 1.99 \text{ or } \dfrac{2 \text{ mg}}{\text{day}}$

$\dfrac{2 \text{ mg}}{\text{day}} \bigg| \dfrac{0.6 \text{ mL}}{15 \text{ mg}} \bigg| \dfrac{2 \times 0.6}{15} \bigg| \dfrac{1.2}{15} = \dfrac{0.08 \text{ mL}}{\text{day}}$

4.
$$\frac{25\ \text{units}}{\text{kg/day}}\left|\frac{1\ \text{kg}}{1000\ \text{g}}\right.\left|\frac{996\ \text{g}}{2\ \text{doses}}\right.\left|\text{day}\right|\frac{25\times1\times996}{1000\times2}\left|\frac{24{,}900}{2000}\right.=\frac{12.45\ \text{or}\ 12.5\ \text{units}}{\text{dose}}$$

$$\frac{12.5\ \text{units}}{\text{dose}}\left|\frac{\text{mL}}{67\ \text{units}}\right.\left|\frac{12.5}{67}\right.=\frac{0.18\ \text{or}\ 0.2\ \text{mL}}{\text{dose}}$$

5.
$$\frac{5\ \text{mg}}{\text{kg/day}}\left|\frac{1\ \text{kg}}{1000\ \text{g}}\right.\left|\frac{996\ \text{g}}{4\ \text{doses}}\right.\left|\text{day}\right|\frac{5\times1\times996}{1000\times4}\left|\frac{4980}{4000}\right.=\frac{1.24\ \text{or}\ 1.2\ \text{mg}}{\text{dose}}$$

$$\frac{1.2\ \text{mg}}{\text{dose}}\left|\frac{\text{mL}}{10\ \text{mg}}\right.\left|\frac{1.2}{10}\right.=\frac{0.12\ \text{or}\ 0.1\ \text{mL}}{\text{dose}}$$

Case Study 19: Cerebral Palsy

Orders requiring calculations: Lactulose 3 g PO tid; Depakote 30 mg/kg/day PO in three divided doses; diazepam 2.5 mg PO daily; chlorothiazide 250 mg PO daily; Dilantin 5 mg/kg/day PO in three divided doses

1.
$$\frac{3\ \text{g}}{10\ \text{g}}\left|\frac{15\ \text{mL}}{10}\right.\left|\frac{3\times15}{10}\right.\left|\frac{45}{10}\right.=4.5\ \text{or}\ 5\ \text{mL}$$

2.
$$\frac{30\ \text{mg}}{\text{kg/day}}\left|\frac{38\ \text{kg}}{3\ \text{doses}}\right.\left|\text{day}\right|\frac{30\times38}{3}\left|\frac{1140}{3}\right.=\frac{380\ \text{mg}}{\text{dose}}$$

$$\frac{380\ \text{mg}}{125\ \text{mg}}\left|\frac{\text{tablet}}{125}\right.\left|\frac{380}{125}\right.=3.04\ \text{or}\ 3\ \text{tablets}$$

3.
$$\frac{2.5\ \text{mg}}{5\ \text{mg}}\left|\frac{\text{tablet}}{5}\right.\left|\frac{2.5}{5}\right.=0.5\ \text{tablet}$$

4.
$$\frac{250\ \text{mg}}{250\ \text{mg}}\left|\frac{\text{tablet}}{250}\right.\left|\frac{250}{250}\right.=1\ \text{tablet}$$

5.
$$\frac{5\ \text{mg}}{\text{kg/day}}\left|\frac{38\ \text{kg}}{3\ \text{dose}}\right.\left|\text{day}\right|\frac{5\ \text{mL}}{125\ \text{mg}}\left|\frac{5\times38\times5}{3\times125}\right.\left|\frac{950}{375}\right.=\frac{2.53\ \text{or}\ 2.5\ \text{mL}}{\text{dose}}$$

Case Study 20: Hyperbilirubinemia

Orders requiring calculations: Albumin 5% infusion 1 g/kg 1 hr before exchange; ampicillin 100 mg/kg/dose IV every 12h; gentamicin 2.5 mg/kg/dose IV every 12h; 120 mL/kg/day formula; IV D10W 120 mL/kg/day

1.
$$\frac{1\ \text{g}}{\text{kg}}\left|\frac{1\ \text{kg}}{1000\ \text{g}}\right.\left|\frac{2210\ \text{g}}{}\right.\left|\frac{1\times1\times221}{100}\right.\left|\frac{221}{100}\right.=2.21\ \text{or}\ 2.2\ \text{g}$$

2.
$$\frac{100\ \text{mg}}{\text{kg/dose}}\left|\frac{1\ \text{kg}}{1000\ \text{g}}\right.\left|\frac{2210\ \text{g}}{}\right.\left|\frac{1\times221}{1}\right.\left|\frac{221}{1}\right.=\frac{221\ \text{mg}}{\text{dose}}$$

$$\frac{221\ \text{mg}}{250\ \text{mg}}\left|\frac{5\ \text{mL}}{250}\right.\left|\frac{221\times5}{250}\right.\left|\frac{1105}{250}\right.=4.42\ \text{or}\ 4.4\ \text{mL}$$

3.
$$\frac{4\ \text{mg}}{\text{kg/dose}}\left|\frac{1\ \text{kg}}{1000\ \text{g}}\right.\left|\frac{2210\ \text{g}}{}\right.\left|\frac{4\times1\times221}{100}\right.\left|\frac{884}{100}\right.=\frac{8.84\ \text{or}\ 8.8\ \text{mg}}{\text{dose}}$$

$$\frac{8.8\ \text{mg}}{2\ \text{mg}}\left|\frac{\text{mL}}{2}\right.\left|\frac{8.8}{2}\right.=4.4\ \text{mL}$$

4.
$$\frac{120\ \text{mL}}{\text{kg/day}}\left|\frac{1\ \text{kg}}{1000\ \text{g}}\right.\left|\frac{2210\ \text{g}}{}\right.\left|\frac{12\times1\times221}{10}\right.\left|\frac{2652}{10}\right.=\frac{265.2\ \text{or}\ 265\ \text{mL}}{\text{day}}$$

5.
$$\frac{120\ \text{mL}}{\text{kg/day}}\left|\frac{1\ \text{kg}}{1000\ \text{g}}\right.\left|\frac{2210\ \text{g}}{24\ \text{hr}}\right.\left|\text{day}\right|\frac{12\times1\times221}{10\times24}\left|\frac{2652}{240}\right.=\frac{11.05\ \text{or}\ 11\ \text{mL}}{\text{hr}}$$

Case Study 21: Spontaneous Abortion

Orders requiring calculations: Rhogam 300 mcg IM; IV D5/0.9% NS at 100 mL/hr; oxytocin (Pitocin) 10 units infused at 20 mL/min; meperidine 50 mg IM every 4h; ibuprofen 400 mg PO

1.
$$\frac{300\ \text{mcg}}{}\left|\frac{1\ \text{ml}}{300\ \text{mcg}}\right.\left|\frac{1}{}\right.=1\ \text{mL}$$

2.
$$\frac{100\ \text{mL}}{\text{hr}}\left|\frac{15\ \text{gtt}}{\text{mL}}\right.\left|\frac{1\ \text{hr}}{60\ \text{min}}\right.\left|\frac{10\times15\times1}{6}\right.\left|\frac{150}{6}\right.=\frac{25\ \text{gtt}}{\text{min}}$$

3.
$$\frac{20\ \text{mU}}{\text{min}}\left|\frac{500\ \text{ml}}{10\ \text{U}}\right.\left|\frac{1\ \text{U}}{1000\ \text{mU}}\right.\left|\frac{60\ \text{min}}{1\ \text{hr}}\right.\left|\frac{2\times5\times1\times6}{1\times1\times1}\right.\left|\frac{60}{1}\right.=\frac{60\ \text{mL}}{\text{hr}}$$

4. $\dfrac{50 \ \text{mg} \ \bigg| \ \fbox{mL} \ \bigg| \ 5}{100 \ \text{mg} \ | \ 10} = 0.5 \ \text{mL}$

5. $\dfrac{400 \ \text{mg} \ \bigg| \ \fbox{tablet} \ \bigg| \ 4}{200 \ \text{mg} \ | \ 2} = 2 \ \text{tablets}$

Case Study 22: Bipolar Disorder

Orders requiring calculations: IV 0.9% NS at 75 mL/hr; lithium 300 mg, lithium 300 mg; clonazepam 0.5 mg; clonazepam 1 mg; doxepin 25 mg

1. $\dfrac{75 \ \text{mL} \ \bigg| \ 20 \ \text{gtt} \ \bigg| \ 1 \ \text{hr} \ \bigg| \ 75 \times 2 \times 1 \ \bigg| \ 150}{\text{hr} \ \bigg| \ \text{mL} \ \bigg| \ 60 \ \text{min} \ \bigg| \ 6 \ \bigg| \ 6} = \dfrac{25 \ \text{gtt}}{\text{min}}$

2. $\dfrac{300 \ \text{mg} \ \bigg| \ \fbox{capsule} \ \bigg| \ 30}{150 \ \text{mg} \ | \ 15} = 2 \ \text{capsules}$

3. $\dfrac{0.5 \ \text{mg} \ \bigg| \ \fbox{tablet} \ \bigg| \ 0.5}{0.5 \ \text{mg} \ | \ 0.5} = 1 \ \text{tablet}$

4. $\dfrac{1 \ \text{mg} \ \bigg| \ \fbox{tablet} \ \bigg| \ 1}{0.5 \ \text{mg} \ | \ 0.5} = 2 \ \text{tablets}$

5. $\dfrac{50 \ \text{mg} \ \bigg| \ \fbox{tablet} \ \bigg| \ 50}{25 \ \text{mg} \ | \ 25} = 2 \ \text{tablets}$

Case Study 23: Anorexia Nervosa

Orders requiring calculations: IV 1000 mL/8 hr; olanzapine (Zyprexa) 10 mg; fluoxetine (Prozac) 60 mg/day; Amitriptyline 25 mg; Cyproheptadine 32 mg/day

1. $\dfrac{1000 \ \fbox{mL}}{8 \ \fbox{hr}} = \dfrac{125 \ \text{mL}}{\text{hr}}$

2. $\dfrac{10 \ \text{mg} \ \bigg| \ \fbox{tablets} \ \bigg| \ 10}{5 \ \text{mg} \ | \ 5} = 2 \ \text{tablets}$

3. $\dfrac{60 \ \text{mg} \ \bigg| \ 5 \ \fbox{mL} \ \bigg| \ 6 \times 5 \ \bigg| \ 30}{20 \ \text{mg} \ \bigg| \ 2 \ \bigg| \ 2} = 15 \ \text{mL}$

4. $\dfrac{25 \ \text{mg} \ \bigg| \ 5 \ \fbox{mL} \ \bigg| \ 25 \times 5 \ \bigg| \ 125}{10 \ \text{mg} \ \bigg| \ 10 \ \bigg| \ 10} = 12.5 \ \text{mL}$

5. $\dfrac{32 \ \fbox{mg} \ \bigg| \ \text{day}}{\text{day} \ \bigg| \ 4 \ \fbox{doses}} = \dfrac{8 \ \text{mg}}{\text{dose}}$

$\dfrac{8 \ \text{mg} \ \bigg| \ 5 \ \fbox{mL} \ \bigg| \ 8 \times 5 \ \bigg| \ 40}{2 \ \text{mg} \ \bigg| \ 2 \ \bigg| \ 2} = 20 \ \text{mL}$

Case Study 24: Clinical Depression

Orders requiring calculations: IV 100 mL/hr; glycopyrrolate (Robinul) 4.4 mcg/kg; Zoloft 50 mg PO every AM; Sinequan 25 mg PO tid; Parnate 30 mg/day PO in 2 divided doses

1. $\dfrac{100 \ \text{mL} \ \bigg| \ 10 \ \fbox{gtt} \ \bigg| \ 1 \ \text{hr} \ \bigg| \ 10 \times 10 \ \bigg| \ 100}{\text{hr} \ \bigg| \ \text{mL} \ \bigg| \ 60 \ \fbox{min} \ \bigg| \ 6 \ \bigg| \ 6} = \dfrac{16.6 \ \text{or} \ 17 \ \text{gtt}}{\text{min}}$

2. $\dfrac{4.4 \ \text{mcg} \ \bigg| \ \fbox{mL} \ \bigg| \ 1 \ \text{kg} \ \bigg| \ 175 \ \text{lb} \ \bigg| \ 4.4 \times 1 \times 175 \ \bigg| \ 770}{\text{kg} \ \bigg| \ 200 \ \text{mcg} \ \bigg| \ 2.2 \ \text{lb} \ \bigg| \ 200 \times 2.2 \ \bigg| \ 440} = 1.75 \ \text{or} \ 1.8 \ \text{mL}$

3. $\dfrac{50 \ \text{mg} \ \bigg| \ \fbox{tablet} \ \bigg| \ 5}{50 \ \text{mg} \ | \ 5} = 1 \ \text{tablet}$

4. $\dfrac{25 \ \text{mg} \ \bigg| \ \fbox{capsule} \ \bigg| \ 25}{25 \ \text{mg} \ | \ 25} = 1 \ \text{capsule}$

5. $\dfrac{30 \ \fbox{mg} \ \bigg| \ \text{day} \ \bigg| \ 30}{\text{day} \ \bigg| \ 2 \ \fbox{doses} \ \bigg| \ 2} = \dfrac{15 \ \text{mg}}{\text{dose}}$

$\dfrac{15 \ \text{mg} \ \bigg| \ \fbox{tablet} \ \bigg| \ 15}{10 \ \text{mg} \ | \ 10} = 1.5 \ \text{tablets}$

Case Study 25: Alzheimer's Disease

Orders requiring calculations: IV 1000 mL/8 hr; donepezil (Aricept) 5 mg; thioridazine (Mellaril) 25 mg; imipramine (Tofranil) 50 mg; temazepam (Restoril) 7.5 mg

1.
$$\frac{1000 \text{ mL}}{8 \text{ hr}} \cdot \frac{10 \text{ gtt}}{\text{mL}} \cdot \frac{1 \text{ hr}}{60 \text{ min}} \cdot \frac{100 \times 10 \times 1}{8 \times 6} \cdot \frac{1000}{48} = \frac{20.83 \text{ or } 21 \text{ gtt}}{\text{min}}$$

2.
$$\frac{5 \text{ mg}}{5 \text{ mg}} \cdot \frac{\text{tablet}}{} \cdot \frac{5}{5} = 1 \text{ tablet}$$

3.
$$\frac{25 \text{ mg}}{25 \text{ mg}} \cdot \frac{\text{tablet}}{} \cdot \frac{25}{25} = 1 \text{ tablet}$$

4.
$$\frac{50 \text{ mg}}{25 \text{ mg}} \cdot \frac{\text{tablet}}{} \cdot \frac{50}{25} = 2 \text{ tablets}$$

5.
$$\frac{7.5 \text{ mg}}{15 \text{ mg}} \cdot \frac{\text{tablet}}{} \cdot \frac{7.5}{15} = 0.5 \text{ tablet}$$

Case Study 26: Otitis Media

Orders requiring calculations: Amoxicillin 45/kg/day, Acetaminophen 120 mg, Ibuprofen 5 mg/kg, Zyrtec 2.5 mg, Pedialyte 75 mL/kg

1.
$$\frac{45 \text{ mg}}{\text{kg/day}} \cdot \frac{5 \text{ mL}}{125 \text{ mg}} \cdot \frac{\text{day}}{2 \text{ doses}} \cdot \frac{1 \text{ kg}}{2.2 \text{ lb}} \cdot \frac{23 \text{ lb}}{} \cdot \frac{45 \times 5 \times 1 \times 23}{125 \times 2 \times 2.2} \cdot \frac{5175}{550} = \frac{9.4 \text{ or } 9 \text{ mL}}{\text{dose}}$$

2.
$$\frac{120 \text{ mg}}{100 \text{ mg}} \cdot \frac{\text{mL}}{10} \cdot \frac{12}{10} = 1.2 \text{ or } 1 \text{ mL}$$

3.
$$\frac{5 \text{ mg}}{\text{kg}} \cdot \frac{5 \text{ mL}}{100 \text{ mg}} \cdot \frac{1 \text{ kg}}{2.2 \text{ lb}} \cdot \frac{23 \text{ lb}}{} \cdot \frac{5 \times 5 \times 1 \times 23}{100 \times 2.2} \cdot \frac{575}{220} = 2.6 \text{ or } 3 \text{ mL}$$

4.
$$\frac{2.5 \text{ mg}}{1 \text{ mg}} \cdot \frac{\text{mL}}{1} \cdot \frac{2.5}{1} = 2.5 \text{ or } 3 \text{ mL}$$

5.
$$\frac{75 \text{ mL}}{\text{kg/8 hr}} \cdot \frac{1 \text{ kg}}{2.2 \text{ lb}} \cdot \frac{23 \text{ lb}}{} \cdot \frac{75 \times 1 \times 23}{8 \times 2.2} \cdot \frac{1725}{17.6} = \frac{98 \text{ mL}}{\text{hr}}$$

Case Study 27: Seizures

Orders requiring calculations: IV D5W/0.45% NS, Dilantin 2 mg/kg/min, Diazepam 0.3/kg, Acetaminophen 320 mg, Ibuprofen 7.5 mg/kg

1.
$$\frac{500 \text{ mL}}{8 \text{ hr}} \cdot \frac{500}{8} = \frac{62.5 \text{ or } 63 \text{ mL}}{\text{hr}}$$

2.
$$\frac{2 \text{ mg}}{\text{kg/15 min}} \cdot \frac{50 \text{ mL}}{100 \text{ mg}} \cdot \frac{1 \text{ kg}}{2.2 \text{ lb}} \cdot \frac{60 \text{ lb}}{1 \text{ hr}} \cdot \frac{60 \text{ min}}{} \cdot \frac{2 \times 50 \times 6 \times 6}{15 \times 1 \times 2.2} \cdot \frac{3600}{33} = \frac{109 \text{ mL}}{\text{hr}}$$

3.
$$\frac{0.3 \text{ mg}}{\text{kg}} \cdot \frac{\text{mL}}{5 \text{ mg}} \cdot \frac{1 \text{ kg}}{2.2 \text{ lb}} \cdot \frac{60 \text{ lb}}{} \cdot \frac{0.3 \times 1 \times 60}{5 \times 2.2} \cdot \frac{18}{11} = 1.63 \text{ or } 1.6 \text{ mL}$$

4.
$$\frac{320 \text{ mg}}{100 \text{ mg}} \cdot \frac{\text{mL}}{10} \cdot \frac{32}{10} = 3.2 \text{ or } 3 \text{ mL}$$

5.
$$\frac{7.5 \text{ mg}}{\text{kg}} \cdot \frac{5 \text{ mL}}{100 \text{ mg}} \cdot \frac{1 \text{ kg}}{2.2 \text{ lb}} \cdot \frac{60 \text{ lb}}{} \cdot \frac{7.5 \times 5 \times 1 \times 6}{10 \times 2.2} \cdot \frac{225}{22} = 10.2 \text{ or } 10 \text{ mL}$$

Case Study 28: Fever of Unknown Origin

Orders requiring calculations: Acetaminophen 400 mg, Ibuprofen 7.5 mg/kg, IV D5W/0.45% NS mL/hr and gtt/min, Unasyn 1500 mg

1.
$$\frac{400 \text{ mg}}{500 \text{ mg}} \cdot \frac{15 \text{ mL}}{5} \cdot \frac{4 \times 15}{5} \cdot \frac{60}{5} = 12 \text{ mL}$$

2.
$$\frac{7.5 \text{ mg}}{\text{kg}} \cdot \frac{5 \text{ mL}}{100 \text{ mg}} \cdot \frac{1 \text{ kg}}{2.2 \text{ lb}} \cdot \frac{80 \text{ lb}}{} \cdot \frac{7.5 \times 5 \times 1 \times 8}{10 \times 2.2} \cdot \frac{300}{22} = 13.6 \text{ or } 14 \text{ mL}$$

3.
$$\frac{500 \text{ mL}}{4 \text{ hr}} \cdot \frac{500}{4} = \frac{125 \text{ mL}}{\text{hr}}$$

4.
$$\frac{500 \text{ mL}}{4 \text{ hr}} \cdot \frac{1 \text{ hr}}{60 \text{ min}} \cdot \frac{60 \text{ gtt}}{\text{mL}} \cdot \frac{500 \times 1}{4} \cdot \frac{500}{4} = \frac{125 \text{ gtt}}{\text{min}}$$

5.
$$\frac{1500 \text{ mg}}{30 \text{ min}} \cdot \frac{50 \text{ mL}}{1.5 \text{ g}} \cdot \frac{1 \text{ g}}{1000 \text{ mg}} \cdot \frac{60 \text{ min}}{1 \text{ hr}} \cdot \frac{15 \times 5 \times 6}{3 \times 1.5 \times 1} \cdot \frac{450}{4.5} = \frac{100 \text{ mL}}{\text{hr}}$$

Case Study 29: TURP with CBI

Orders requiring calculations: IV D5W/.45% NS in mL/hr and gtt/min, Cipro 400 mg, Colace 100 mg, dimenhydrinate 25 mg

1. $\dfrac{1000 \;\boxed{mL}}{8\,\boxed{hr}} \bigg| \dfrac{1000}{8} = \dfrac{125}{hr}\; mL$

2. $\dfrac{1000 \;\cancel{mL}}{8\;\cancel{hr}} \bigg| \dfrac{2\theta\;\boxed{gtt}}{\cancel{mL}} \bigg| \dfrac{1\,\cancel{hr}}{6\theta\;\boxed{min}} \bigg| \dfrac{1000 \times 2 \times 1}{8 \times 6} \bigg| \dfrac{2000}{48} = \dfrac{41.6 \text{ or } 42}{min}\; gtt$

3. $\dfrac{4\theta\theta\;\cancel{mg}}{6\theta\;\cancel{min}} \bigg| \dfrac{200\;\boxed{mL}}{4\theta\theta\;\cancel{mg}} \bigg| \dfrac{6\theta\;\cancel{min}}{1\,\boxed{hr}} \bigg| \dfrac{200}{1} = \dfrac{200}{hr}\; mL$

4. $\dfrac{100\;\cancel{mg}}{} \bigg| \dfrac{\boxed{capsule}}{100\;\cancel{mg}} \bigg| \dfrac{100}{100} = 1 \text{ capsule}$

5. $\dfrac{25\;\cancel{mg}}{} \bigg| \dfrac{\boxed{mL}}{50\;\cancel{mg}} \bigg| \dfrac{25}{50} = 0.5 \text{ mL}$

Case Study 30: Hypercholesterolemia

Orders requiring calculations: Chantix 0.5 mg for days 1–8, Lipitor 20 mg, cholestyramine resin 4 g, niacin 1.5 g/day

1. $\dfrac{0.5\;\cancel{mg}}{} \bigg| \dfrac{\boxed{tablet}}{0.5\;\cancel{mg}} \bigg| \dfrac{0.5}{0.5} = 1 \text{ tablet}$

2. $\dfrac{1\;\cancel{mg}}{} \bigg| \dfrac{\boxed{tablet}}{0.5\;\cancel{mg}} \bigg| \dfrac{1}{0.5} = 2 \text{ tablets}$

3. $\dfrac{2\theta\;\cancel{mg}}{} \bigg| \dfrac{\boxed{tablets}}{1\theta\;\cancel{mg}} \bigg| \dfrac{2}{1} = 2 \text{ tablets}$

4. $\dfrac{4\,\boxed{g}}{\cancel{dose}} \bigg| \dfrac{2\;\cancel{doses}}{\boxed{day}} \bigg| \dfrac{4 \times 2}{} \bigg| \dfrac{8}{} = \dfrac{8}{day}\; g$

5. $\dfrac{1.5 \text{ g}}{\boxed{day}} \bigg| \dfrac{\boxed{tablet}}{5\theta\theta\;\cancel{mg}} \bigg| \dfrac{100\theta\;\cancel{mg}}{1 \text{ g}} \bigg| \dfrac{1.5 \times 10}{5 \times 1} \bigg| \dfrac{15}{5} = \dfrac{3 \text{ tablets}}{day}$

Case Study 31: Hypertension

Orders requiring calculations: mL/meal of fluids, nifedipine 60 mg, Colace 100 mg, hydrochlorothiazide 25 mg, Weight gain

1. $\dfrac{2\;\cancel{L}}{\cancel{day}} \bigg| \dfrac{\cancel{day}}{3\;\boxed{meals}} \bigg| \dfrac{1000\;\boxed{mL}}{1\;\cancel{L}} \bigg| \dfrac{2 \times 1000}{3 \times 1} \bigg| \dfrac{2000}{3} = \dfrac{666.6 \text{ or } 667}{meal}\; mL$

2. $\dfrac{6\theta\;\cancel{mg}}{} \bigg| \dfrac{\boxed{tablet}}{3\theta\;\cancel{mg}} \bigg| \dfrac{6}{3} = 2 \text{ tablets}$

3. $\dfrac{100\;\cancel{mg}}{} \bigg| \dfrac{\boxed{capsule}}{100\;\cancel{mg}} \bigg| \dfrac{100}{100} = 1 \text{ capsule}$

4. $\dfrac{25\;\cancel{mg}}{} \bigg| \dfrac{\boxed{tablet}}{50\;\cancel{mg}} \bigg| \dfrac{25}{50} = 0.5 \text{ tablet}$

5. $\dfrac{5\;\cancel{kg}}{} \bigg| \dfrac{2.2\;\boxed{lb}}{1\;\cancel{kg}} \bigg| \dfrac{5 \times 2.2}{1} \bigg| \dfrac{11}{1} = 11 \text{ lb}$

Case Study 32: Diabetic Ketoacidosis

Orders requiring calculations: IV 0.9% NS 20 mL/kg/hr, regular insulin 0.15 units/kg, regular insulin 0.1 unit/kg/hr, IV D5W/0.45% NS, ampicillin sodium 500 mg

1. $\dfrac{1000\;\boxed{mL}}{8\,\boxed{hr}} \bigg| \dfrac{1000}{8} = \dfrac{125}{hr}\; mL$

2. $\dfrac{0.15\;\cancel{units}}{\cancel{kg}} \bigg| \dfrac{25\theta\;\boxed{mL}}{25\theta\;\cancel{units}} \bigg| \dfrac{1\;\cancel{kg}}{2.2\;\cancel{lb}} \bigg| \dfrac{125\;\cancel{lb}}{} \bigg| \dfrac{0.15 \times 1 \times 125}{2.2} \bigg| \dfrac{18.75}{2.2} = 8.52 \text{ or } 8.5 \text{ mL}$

3. $\dfrac{0.1\;\cancel{unit}}{\cancel{kg}/\boxed{hr}} \bigg| \dfrac{25\theta\;\boxed{mL}}{25\theta\;\cancel{units}} \bigg| \dfrac{1\;\cancel{kg}}{2.2\;\cancel{lb}} \bigg| \dfrac{125\;\cancel{lb}}{} \bigg| \dfrac{0.1 \times 1 \times 125}{2.2} \bigg| \dfrac{12.5}{2.2} = \dfrac{5.68 \text{ or } 5.7}{hr}\; mL$

4. $\dfrac{10\;\boxed{mL}}{\cancel{kg}/\boxed{hr}} \bigg| \dfrac{1\;\cancel{kg}}{2.2\;\cancel{lb}} \bigg| \dfrac{125\;\cancel{lb}}{} \bigg| \dfrac{10 \times 1 \times 125}{2.2} \bigg| \dfrac{1250}{2.2} = \dfrac{568.1 \text{ or } 568}{hr}\; mL$

5. $\dfrac{5\theta\theta\;\cancel{mg}}{3\theta\;\cancel{min}} \bigg| \dfrac{10\theta\;\boxed{mL}}{1\;\cancel{g}} \bigg| \dfrac{1\;\cancel{g}}{100\theta\;\cancel{mg}} \bigg| \dfrac{6\theta\;\cancel{min}}{1\,\boxed{hr}} \bigg| \dfrac{5 \times 10 \times 6}{3 \times 1 \times 1} \bigg| \dfrac{300}{3} = \dfrac{100}{hr}\; mL$

Case Study 33: End–Stage Renal Failure

Orders requiring calculations: Furosemide 120 mg, Zaroxolyn 10 mg, Vasotec 2.5 mg, Epogen 100 units/kg, Calcium Carbonate 10 g/day

1. $\dfrac{120 \text{ mg}}{80 \text{ mg}} \bigg| \dfrac{\text{tablet}}{} \bigg| \dfrac{12}{8} = 1.5$ tablets

2. $\dfrac{10 \text{ mg}}{5 \text{ mg}} \bigg| \dfrac{\text{tablet}}{} \bigg| \dfrac{10}{5} = 2$ tablets

3. $\dfrac{2.5 \text{ mg}}{2.5 \text{ mg}} \bigg| \dfrac{\text{tablet}}{} \bigg| \dfrac{2.5}{2.5} = 1$ tablet

4. $\dfrac{100 \text{ units}}{\text{kg}} \bigg| \dfrac{\text{mL}}{4000 \text{ units}} \bigg| \dfrac{1 \text{ kg}}{2.2 \text{ lb}} \bigg| \dfrac{140 \text{ lb}}{} \bigg| \dfrac{1 \times 1 \times 14}{4 \times 2.2} \bigg| \dfrac{14}{8.8} = 1.59$ or 1.6 mL

5. $\dfrac{10 \text{ g}}{\text{day}} \bigg| \dfrac{\text{tablet}}{1500 \text{ mg}} \bigg| \dfrac{1000 \text{ mg}}{1 \text{ g}} \bigg| \dfrac{\text{day}}{3 \text{ meals}} \bigg| \dfrac{10 \times 10}{15 \times 1 \times 3} \bigg| \dfrac{100}{45} = \dfrac{2.2 \text{ or } 2 \text{ tablets}}{\text{meals}}$

Case Study 34: Fluid Volume Deficit

Orders requiring calculations: IV 0.9% NS/2.5% Dextrose 50 mL/kg, Acetaminophen 400 mg, Ibuprofen 7.5 mg/kg, mL/hr of PO fluids, mL/hr of Pedialyte

1. $\dfrac{50 \text{ mL}}{\text{kg}/4 \text{ hr}} \bigg| \dfrac{1 \text{ kg}}{2.2 \text{ lb}} \bigg| \dfrac{35 \text{ lb}}{} \bigg| \dfrac{50 \times 1 \times 35}{4 \times 2.2} \bigg| \dfrac{1750}{8.8} = 198.8$ or $199 \dfrac{\text{mL}}{\text{hr}}$

2. $\dfrac{400 \text{ mg}}{100 \text{ mg}} \bigg| \dfrac{\text{mL}}{1} \bigg| \dfrac{4}{} = 4$ mL

3. $\dfrac{7.5 \text{ mg}}{\text{kg}} \bigg| \dfrac{5 \text{ mL}}{100 \text{ mg}} \bigg| \dfrac{1 \text{ kg}}{2.2 \text{ lb}} \bigg| \dfrac{35 \text{ lb}}{} \bigg| \dfrac{7.5 \times 5 \times 1 \times 35}{100 \times 2.2} \bigg| \dfrac{1312.5}{220} = 5.9$ or 6 mL

4. $\dfrac{1.5 \text{ oz}}{\text{lb}/24 \text{ hr}} \bigg| \dfrac{30 \text{ mL}}{1 \text{ oz}} \bigg| \dfrac{35 \text{ lb}}{} \bigg| \dfrac{1.5 \times 30 \times 35}{24 \times 1} \bigg| \dfrac{1575}{24} = 65.6$ or $66 \dfrac{\text{mL}}{\text{hr}}$

5. $\dfrac{53 \text{ oz}}{24 \text{ hr}} \bigg| \dfrac{30 \text{ mL}}{1 \text{ oz}} \bigg| \dfrac{53 \times 30}{24 \times 1} \bigg| \dfrac{1590}{24} = 66.2$ or $66 \dfrac{\text{mL}}{\text{hr}}$

Case Study 35: Increased Intracranial Pressure

Orders requiring calculations: IV 0.9% NS, Dilantin 10 mg/kg, Mannitol 0.25 g/kg, Dexamethasone 10 mg, Furosemide 0.5 mg/kg

1. $\dfrac{1000 \text{ mL}}{10 \text{ hr}} \bigg| \dfrac{1000}{10} = \dfrac{100 \text{ mL}}{\text{hr}}$

2. $\dfrac{10 \text{ mg}}{\text{Kg}} \bigg| \dfrac{20 \text{ mL}}{1000 \text{ mg}} \bigg| \dfrac{75 \text{ kg}}{} \bigg| \dfrac{1 \times 2 \times 75}{10} \bigg| \dfrac{150}{10} = 15$ mL

3. $\dfrac{0.25 \text{ g}}{\text{Kg}/\text{hr}} \bigg| \dfrac{500 \text{ mL}}{100 \text{ g}} \bigg| \dfrac{75 \text{ kg}}{} \bigg| \dfrac{0.25 \times 5 \times 75}{1} \bigg| \dfrac{93.7}{1} = 93.7$ or $94 \dfrac{\text{mL}}{\text{hr}}$

4. $\dfrac{10 \text{ mg}}{120 \text{ mg}} \bigg| \dfrac{5 \text{ mL}}{12} \bigg| \dfrac{1 \times 5}{12} \bigg| \dfrac{5}{} = 0.41$ or 0.4 mL

5. $\dfrac{0.5 \text{ mg}}{\text{Kg}} \bigg| \dfrac{\text{mL}}{10 \text{ mg}} \bigg| \dfrac{75 \text{ kg}}{} \bigg| \dfrac{0.5 \times 75}{10} \bigg| \dfrac{37.5}{10} = 3.75$ or 3.7 mL

Comprehensive Post-Test

Comprehensive Post-Test

Name _____   **Date** _____

1. Order: Lopressor 12.5 mg PO daily for severe heart failure.

   Supply: Lopressor 25 mg/tablets

   ▶ **How many tablets will you give?** _____

2. Order: Synthroid 0.2 mg PO daily for hypothyroidism.

   Supply: Synthroid 200 mcg/tablets

   ▶ **How many tablets will you give?** _____

3. Order: Micro K 30 mEq PO daily for hypokalemia.

   Supply: Micro K 10 mEq/capsules

   ▶ **How many capsules will you give?** _____

4. Order: Phenergan 12.5 mg IV every 4 hours for nausea.

   Supply: Phenergan 25 mg/mL

   ▶ **How many milliliters will you give?** _____

5. Order: 1000 mL of D5W/0.45 NS to infuse over 12 hours

   Drop factor: 15 gtt/mL

   ▶ **Calculate the number of drops per minute.** _____

6. Order: Heparin 2500 units/hr IV for thrombophlebitis.

   Supply: Heparin 25,000 units/500 mL

   ▶ **Calculate milliliter per hour to set the
   IV pump.** _____

7. Order: Infuse Heparin at 45 mL/hr IV for thrombophlebitis.

   Supply: Heparin 25,000 units/500 mL

   ▶ **How many units per hour is the
   patient receiving?** _____

8. Order: Infuse 250 mL bolus of 0.9% NS at 33 gtt/min

   Supply: 250 mL 0.9% NS with 20 gtt/mL tubing

   ▶ **How many hours will it take to infuse the
   IV bolus?** _____

(Post-Test continues on page 260)

9. Order: Pentamidine: 4 mg/kg IV daily for 14 days for patient weighing 130 lb for severe Pneumocystis carinii pneumonia.

Supply: Pentamidine 300 mg/250 mL D5W to infuse over 60 min.

▶ **Calculate the milliliters per hour to set the IV pump.** _____

10. Order: Naloxone (Narcan) 0.01 mg/kg IV for narcotic overdose for child weighing 35 kg.

Supply: Naloxone (Narcan) 0.4 mg/mL

▶ **How many milliliters will you give?** _____

11. Order: Epogen 150 units/kg SQ three times weekly due to anemia secondary to chemotherapy for a patient weighing 80 kg.

Supply: Epogen 20,000 units/mL

▶ **How many milliliters will you give?** _____

12. Order: Acyclovir 5 mg/kg IV every 8 hours for 7 days for cutaneous herpes simplex for a patient weighing 70 kg.

Supply: Acyclovir 1-g vial

Nursing drug reference: Reconstitute each 1-g vial with 10 mL of sterile water and further dilute in 100 mL 0.9% NS and infuse over 1 hour.

▶ **How many milliliters will you draw from the vial after reconstitution?** _____

▶ **Calculate the milliliters per hour to set the IV pump.** _____

▶ **Calculate the drops per minute with a drop factor of 20 gtt/mL.** _____

13. Order: Vancomycin 1 g IV every 12 hours for severe staphylococcal infection.

Supply: Vancomycin 5-g vial

Nursing drug reference: Reconstitute each 5-g vial with 10 mL of sterile water and further dilute in 250 mL of D5W and infuse over 60 minutes.

▶ **How many milliliters will you draw from the vial after reconstitution?** _____

▶ **Calculate the milliliters per hour to set the IV pump.** _____

▶ **Calculate the drops per minute with a drop factor of 10 gtt/mL.** _____

14. Order: Regular Insulin 8 units/hours for hyperglycemia

    Supply: Regular Insulin 100 units/250 mL 0.9% NS

    ▶ **Calculate milliliters per hours to set the IV pump.** _____

15. Order: Nitroprusside 0.8 mcg/kg/min for hypertensive crisis.

    Supply: Nitroprusside 50 mg/500 mL D5W

    The patient weighs: 143 lb

    ▶ **Calculate milliliters per hour to set the IV pump.** _____

16. Order: Mycostatin oral suspension 500,000 units swish/swallow for oral candidiasis.

    Supply: Mycostatin 100,000 units/mL

    ▶ **How many teaspoons will you give?** _____

17. Order: Dilaudid 140 mL/hr

    Supply: Dilaudid 30 mg/1000 mL D5/NS

    ▶ **Calculate milligrams per hour the patient is receiving.** _____

18. Order: Aminophylline 44 mg/hr for status asthmaticus.

    Supply: Aminophylline 1 g/250 mL D5W

    ▶ **Calculate milliliters per hour to set the IV pump.** _____

19. Order: 1000 mL NS to infuse at 60 gtt/min

    Drop factor: 15 gtt/mL

    ▶ **Calculate how many hours it will take for the IV to infuse.** _____

20. Order: Dopamine (Intropin) 5 mcg/kg/min IV for cardiogenic shock secondary to myocardial infarction.

    Supply: Dopamine 200 mg/250 mL D5W

    ▶ **Calculate the milliliters per hour to set the IV pump.** _____

APPENDIX

Educational Theory of Dimensional Analysis

Dimensional analysis is a problem-solving method based on the principles of cognitive theory. Bruner (1960) theorized that learning is dependent on how information is structured, organized, and conceptualized. He proposed a cognitive learning model that emphasized the acquisition, organization (structure), understanding, and transfer of knowledge—focusing on "how" to learn, rather than "what" to learn. Learning involves associations established according to the principles of continuity and repetition.

Dimensional analysis (also called factor-label method, conversion-factor method, units analysis, and quantity calculus) provides a systematic way to set up problems and helps to organize and evaluate data. Hein (1983) emphasized that dimensional analysis gives a clear understanding of the principles of the problem-solving method that correlates with the ability to verbalize what steps are taken leading to critical thinking. He described dimensional analysis as a useful method for solving a variety of chemistry, physics, mathematics, and daily life problems. He identified that dimensional analysis is often the problem-solving method of choice because it provides a straightforward way to set up problems, gives a clear understanding of the principles of the problem, helps the learner to organize and evaluate data, and assists in identifying errors if the setup of the problem is incorrect.

Goodstein (1983) described dimensional analysis as a problem-solving method that is very simple to understand, reduces errors, and requires less conceptual reasoning power to understand than does the ratio–proportion method. She expressed that "even though the ratio–proportion method was at one time the primary problem-solving method, it has been largely replaced by a dimensional analysis approach in most introductory chemistry textbooks . . . this method condenses multi-step problems into one orderly extended solution."

Peters (1986) identified dimensional analysis as a method used for solving not only chemistry problems but also a variety of other mathematical problems that require conversions. He defined dimensional analysis as a method that can be used whenever two quantities are directly proportional to each other and one quantity must be converted to the other using a conversion factor or conversion relationship.

Literature that has examined the quality of higher education and professional education in the United States (National Institute of Education, 1984) recommends that educators increase the emphasis of the intellectual skills of problem solving and critical thinking. Also recommended is an increased emphasis on the mastery of concepts rather than specific facts. Other literature on curriculum revolution in nursing (Bevis, 1988; Lindeman, 1989; Tanner, 1988) recommends that learning not be characterized merely as a change in behavior or the acquisition of facts, but in seeing and *understanding* the significance of the whole. Because it focuses on "how" to learn, rather than "what" to learn, dimensional analysis supports conceptual mastery and higher-level thinking skills that have become the core of the curriculum change that is sweeping through all levels of education and, most importantly, nursing education.

Bibliography

Bevis, E. (1988). New directions for a new age. In National League for Nursing, *Curriculum revolution: Mandate for change* (pp. 27–52). New York: National League for Nursing (Pub. No. 15–2224).

Bruner, J. (1960). *The process of education*. New York: Random House.

Craig, G. (1995). The effects of dimensional analysis on the medication dosage calculation abilities of nursing students. *Nurse Educator, 20*(3), 14–18.

Craig, G. P. (1997). The effectiveness of dimensional analysis as a problem-solving method for medication calculations from the nursing student perspective. Unpublished doctoral dissertation, Drake University, Des Moines, IA.

Goodstein, M. (1983). Reflections upon mathematics in the introductory chemistry course. *Journal of Chemical Education, 60*(8), 665–667.

Hein, M. (1983). *Foundations of chemistry* (4th ed.). Encino, CA: Dickenson Publishing Company.

Lindeman, C. (1989). Curriculum revolution: Reconceptualizing clinical nursing education. *Nursing and Health Care, 10*(1), 23–28.

National Institute of Education. (1984). *Involvement in learning: Realizing the potential of American higher education*. Washington, DC: National Institute of Education.

Peters, E. (1986). *Introduction to chemical principles* (4th ed.). Saratoga, CA: Saunders College Publishing.

Tanner, C. (1988). Curriculum revolution: The practice mandate. *Nursing and Health Care, 9*(8), 426–430.

Index

A

abacavir (Ziagen), dosage calculation for
  one-factor, 180
  two-factor, 190
abortion, spontaneous, case study of, 233–234
acetaminophen. *see* Tylenol (acetaminophen)
acquired immunodeficiency syndrome (AIDS), case
    study of, 219
acyclovir
  dosage calculation for, two-factor, 132, 188
  IV therapy considerations, 127
adalat (nifedipine), dosage calculation for, one-factor,
    168
administration routes, 66
  enteral, 81–87
  intravenous (*see* intravenous therapy)
  parenteral, 87–93
advil (ibuprofen), dosage calculation for, 71–72
AIDS (acquired immunodeficiency syndrome), case
    study of, 219
Alzheimer's disease, case study of, 237
amikacin (Amikin), dosage calculation for, three-
    factor, 195
aminophylline, dosage calculation for, 199
  IV therapy, 121–123
  three-factor, 155, 161
amiodarone (Cordarone IV), dosage calculation for,
    200
amoxicillin, dosage calculation for, 201
ampicillin. *see* Unasyn (ampicillin)
amrinone, dosage calculation for, three-factor, 154
ancef, dosage calculation for
  three-factor, 149, 196
  two-factor, 118, 136
anemia, sickle cell, case study of, 220
anorexia nervosa, case study of, 235–236
anticoagulants, administration of, 88
apothecaries' measurement system, 32–34
  abbreviations, 31b, 33b
  defined, 32
  other system equivalents for, 38t, 39, 43
  volume in, 32, 33b, 33f, 38t
  weight in, 32, 33b, 33f, 38t

Arabic number system, 6, 6t
  converting between Roman and, 3, 6–9, 18, 21
  defined, 6
ascorbic acid, dosage calculation for, 197
aspirin, dosage calculation for, 70–71
atenolol (Tenormin), dosage calculation for, 200
atropine sulfate, dosage calculation for, 197
  two-factor, 113, 181
  using drug label, 92
augmentin, dosage calculation for
  one-factor, 172
  two-factor, 135
  using drug label, 96
azactam, dosage calculation for, two-factor, 136
azithromycin (Zithromax), dosage calculation for,
    201

B

batch number, of a drug, 75
Benadryl (diphenhydramine), dosage calculation for,
    three-factor, 192
bipolar disorder, case study of, 234–235
bone marrow transplantation, case study of, 221–222
bretylium tosylate, dosage calculation for, three-factor,
    153
bronchopulmonary dysplasia, case study of, 231

C

caplets, administration of, 81, 82f
capsules, administration of, 82, 82f
Celsius temperature, 34
  conversion to Fahrenheit, 36b, 36f, 40, 43–44
ceptaz (ceftazidime), dosage calculation for, two-
    factor, 190
cerebral palsy, case study of, 232
children, medication problems involving, body weight
    and, 112–114, 142–145, 148–150, 154–155,
    157–161
children, medication problems involving, body weight
    and, 180–181, 190–192, 194–196, 201
chronic obstructive pulmonary disease (COPD), case
    study of, 217

265